If The President Had Cancer...

Cancer Care:
How to
find and
get the
best there is.

by
Gary Schine
with Ellen Berlinsky, Ph.D

Sandra Publications • Providence, Rhode Island

Published By:

Allen County Public Library
900 Webster Street
PO Box 2270
Fort Wayne, IN 46801-2270

Sandra Publications
39 Brenton Avenue
Providence, RI 02906

(401)751-3320

To Adam and Laura

ISBN 0-9635824-8-8
Library of Congress Catalog Card Number 93-092558

Printed and bound in the United States of America

❖

Acknowledgments

Many people were helpful to us in bringing this book from an idea to a finished product. We wish to especially acknowledge the help of the following individuals: Maya Rogers, M.D. and Charles Rogers, M.D. for their medical counsel and advice on the manuscript; Roberta Bronson, Maureen Czujak, and Faithe McGrath of the National Library of Medicine for education on the use of NLM databases; Gregg Fredo of the National Cancer Institute's Cancer Information Service for answering our questions about the CIS; Larry Roberts of the *Hartford Courant* for teaching us some of the investigative skills of a professional journalist; Barbara Schermack of the HOPE Center for Life Enhancement, Susan O'Classen, Ralph Perrotta, Tom Policastro, Karen Stern, and Nancy Walz for their advice and counsel; Alan Saven, M.D. of Scripps Clinic and Research Foundation for administering life saving treatment; and last but by no means least, Jeffrey Clark, M.D. of the Roger Williams Cancer Center for his superb follow-up care and for the important information that he provided to us.

Table of Contents

❖

The *He or She* Issue

Unfortunately, the English language does not provide a non-sexist solution to the use of the pronouns *he* and *she*. Traditionally, of course, *he* was used to mean *he* and *she* when not referring to a specific person. Like so many writers, we have been frustrated in trying to find a workable solution to this problem. The overriding concern in writing this book was to provide the information and make it as easy to understand as possible. We also wanted avoid awkward sentence constructions that would serve no purpose other than to accentuate a shortcoming of our language and perhaps to make a political point. Therefore, we have, in many instances, been forced to use the traditional *he* to mean both *he* and *she*.

CHAPTER ONE

❖

Introduction

"You have a lymphoproliferative disorder," the doctor told me. I had no idea what that meant, and the doctor knew it. He was just beginning to break the news to me gently and I guess that was the approach that worked best for him.

As the story unfolded it became clear that my depressed iron level noted at a recent blood drive had nothing to do with poor diet as I had naively surmised. I won't pretend to remember everything that Dr. Telder said at that meeting but I clearly remember a few words like malignancy and leukemia and a few phrases of advice like "make sure your health insurance and life insurance policies are paid up." Mostly I remember thinking about my two year old daughter and my seven year old son growing up without a father and about my wife having to support them, raise them, and explain what happened to Daddy all by herself. "This can't be real," I thought. "I'm only 38; how can I have cancer?" It was very real indeed.

The doctor had a little encouraging news by our next meeting two weeks later. He had completed his diagnostic tests and explained that I had hairy cell leukemia, a rare form of the disease. It could have been worse, in that HCL progresses relatively slowly. "Why I've seen people with HCL live for ten years," he told me. To keep me alive would require major surgery, a splenectomy. That might buy me a few years of relatively trouble free life. Then I might start on a drug called interferon which would manage the illness but not cure it. Interferon comes with sides effects such as periodic flu like symptoms and loss of mental concentration abilities. "There is no cure" the doctor cautioned, "What we want to do is lessen the severity and slow down the progress of the leukemia."

In the meantime my already compromised immune system would deteriorate further, my constant fatigue would get worse, and I might eventually be susceptible to spontaneous external and internal bleeding.

The name "Dr. Telder" is fictitious. Any resemblance to any person's actual name is unintended and coincidental.

1

That was eighteen months ago. Things are different now. This morning I braved the 26 degree cold and ran 2 and 1/2 miles as I do on most mornings. Back then, I had difficulty walking two flights of stairs. I'm working full 8 hour days now. I could easily work more but I don't because I want to spend time with my kids. One thing my experience taught me is how important it is to spend time with them. Last year I could hardly stay awake for eight hours without a nap. My immune system is as capable as it ever was, and spontaneous bleeding is no longer a threat. There is simply no evidence of cancer to be found in my body.

You see, despite Dr. Telder's predictions, I am, by all indications cured of my incurable disease. The doctor simply was unaware of the latest developments in the treatment of HCL. He did not know about two recent treatments that were much more effective than his antiquated treatment proposal of splenectomy followed by interferon.

The treatment that I chose was developed and administered at Scripps Clinic and Research Foundation in LaJolla, California. The treatment, a chemotherapy agent called 2-chlorodeoxyadenosine (2-CDA), involved a seven day intravenous infusion. While the drug had short term side effects like nausea, fever, and flu-like symptoms, there are no known long term side effects. Two weeks after the treatment I returned from California to my home in Rhode Island able to carry on my life, albeit on an abbreviated schedule. Two months after my return I was working full time, exercising for the first time in years, and feeling like a new person. While I have no guarantees, I have been given every reason to believe I will neither suffer a relapse nor later side effects from the treatment.

Once I independently set out to learn about my illness, finding this treatment was not difficult. Through a call to the local chapter of the Leukemia Society of America, I learned that there was a treatment for HCL in clinical trial. A bit of simple research uncovered a technical report about 2-CDA in the venerable *New England Journal of Medicine* and a lay-person summary of the technical report in the equally venerable *Wall Street Journal*. Both articles appeared three months previous to my diagnosis.

Had I not set out to find information on my own, had I not been assertive in seeking and getting the best treatment available, the prognosis offered by Dr. Telder would have been fulfilled.

Every person with a serious illness has the responsibility to be informed about that illness and its treatment options. The seriously ill patient must take responsibility for doing all he can to prolong his life and to strive for the best quality of life possible. As my experience shows, relying solely on one's doctor will not always be adequate. It takes some research and study and some assertiveness to assure that you know what the choices are and to make those choices based on the best information possible.

Some physicians will argue that "a little knowledge is a dangerous thing." To some degree, this argument has merit. However, as my own experience and that of so many others shows, a lack of knowledge can be far more dangerous for a person with a serious illness.

The fact is that not every oncologist can be up to date on the details of the more than 100 kinds of cancer. Developments in medicine come so rapidly that no practitioner could possibly be completely current on every advance in his field. Further, most oncologists have hundreds of patients and do not have the time to research every patient's illness. Patients don't understand this and too often accept their doctor's diagnosis and prognosis without question. They assume the doctor told them all there is to tell. Further, they assume that if there are choices to be made, the doctor is the one to unilaterally make those choices.

Even doctors versed in a particular disease and its treatment options will disagree as to the best course of action. Some are conservative; they prefer to stay with time honored methods rather than risk something new. Others are more aggressive, willing to accept a little risk in the hopes of better results. There is nothing wrong with such differences or with either bias. But you as the patient are the one who should be choosing between the approaches that will have such a profound impact on your life. The only way to make appropriate choices is to gather the best information that you can.

It is comforting to put your full trust and confidence in your physician. However, the ideal of the omniscient doctor and his command of a formidable medical support system is mostly a myth. Doctors are busy people and more than that: they are human. They can not stay on top of every development in their field nor the full spectrum of needs of all their patients all of the time. A patient faced with a serious illness is better served by assuming that he is largely on his own to negotiate the medical system and to find and get the best treatment available.

An editorial in the *New York Times* of December 13, 1992 quotes Dr. Jack Wennberg of the Dartmouth Medical School as saying:

> Doctors often don't know what treatments work and almost surely don't know which treatment best serves their patients.

> *The editorial continues:*
> The choice of medical treatments, it turns out, depends more on folklore than on scientific evidence.

Patients who shift all responsibility for the management of their illness to the doctor contribute to that doctor's already overwhelming burdens. Patients who look to doctors as the highly skilled professionals they are, and not as the all-knowing father figures that they are not, are helping themselves and relieving those doctors from the burden of maintaining the facade of omnipotence.

Taking on some of the responsibility for managing your medical care is important in many ways, not the least being that it is your own life at stake, It goes without saying that your own life is more important to you than to your physician. Therefore, you will be the most motivated to search out the best care available. You are uniquely qualified to make the choices that best fit your needs medically, psychologically, and otherwise. Taking control will also change your perspective on your illness. You will no longer be the passive patient, but rather an active participant in your medical care. This change in perspective will increase your feelings of self worth, making you less like a child and more like a competent adult. Making this change will do much to counter the terror you have felt in coping with your diagnosis of cancer.

Unfortunately, the medical establishment is accustomed to patient compliance. Not all doctors nor other medical professionals look kindly on patients taking responsibility and seeking independent information in the ways that I advocate. You will need to be assertive. But assertiveness without appropriate knowledge is at best ineffective and at worst alienating and counterproductive in a system

4

that thrives on compliance. Assertiveness backed up by information may quite literally mean the difference between life and death.

Clearly my own efforts resulted in a home run; I found a cure for an illness that was supposed to be debilitating and fatal. In my case (at least in retrospect) it was all black and white, there was a bad choice and a much better choice. Not every cancer sufferer will be so fortunate or have choices so clearly contrasted as I did. However, many patients will have choices as to how to battle the formidable enemy called cancer. To know how to make the best choices, indeed to know what the choices are, you need to become informed. You need also to use that information to derive the power you will need to give yourself the best chance possible.

What This Guide Is Meant to Do

Medical science has come a long way in treating cancer. Developments and discoveries continue to come very rapidly. Research and experimentation is constantly taking place at hundreds of hospitals, clinics, and universities throughout the country and the world. It is not unusual for a state of the art treatment to be replaced by a better treatment, and then replaced again by a still better one within a period of several months.

However, people in need often don't get the best care because they are ignorant about their disease and its treatment alternatives. Too many patients assume that their doctor is fully abreast of all the latest information about their condition and its treatment. Further, too many patients are afraid to challenge their doctor's knowledge or his status as the undisputed decision maker.

Because developments come so rapidly, it is simply naive to assume that every doctor is up-to-date on every kind of cancer and treatment. When your life is at stake the fear of challenging or even insulting the doctor by questioning his knowledge or recommendations simply must be overcome.

You must get the best information available and assert your right to make decisions that will impact upon your survival and your quality of life. This guide will show you how to find the information you need to have, how to use it to your advantage, and how to deal with a medical establishment that does not encourage patients to exercise their rights to learn and to decide.

Specifically this guide will show you how to:

❖ *Do Your Own Research*— Even if you are like me with no background or training in medicine, biology, or a related area, you can learn a lot about your illness and treatment options through research. This guide will tell you some of the sources and how to find and use them. It is easy to gather dozens of pages of very current information about your illness and your treatment possibilities. It is not unlikely that you will quickly gather more valuable and current information than your doctor has available, if you follow this guide.

❖ *Ask Your Doctor the Right Questions*— Your doctor, while not your only source of information, is one of your key sources. However, to get the right information. you need to ask the right questions.

❖ *Get a Second Opinion*—Without a second opinion, you can't be sure that the advice you are getting is the best advice, or even good advice. How and where to get a second opinion is covered.

❖ *Find Out about Clinical Trials* — In cancer research, the latest treatments are offered in highly structured and regulated programs called clinical trials. While such trials involve varying degrees of risk, they may be your ticket to prolonging your life. Straightforward steps to finding out about clinical trials are outlined.

❖ *Use Contacts*— In medicine as in most fields, some are more equal than others. Some medical professionals hold prestige and influence; their names will open doors. But you don't necessarily have to be on the inside to use contacts. Chapter six describes how you can get appointments with the doctors who know the most about your particular illness.

❖ *Find Out a Doctor's Qualifications and Abilities*— Too many patients judge doctors based on how nice they are. That's understandable since most patients have no way of judging a doctor's technical competence which, of course, is far more important than his bedside manner. There are easy ways to get information about a doctor's background and increase your chances of retaining a good doctor instead of a mediocre one.

❖ *Anticipate and Overcome Obstacles—* If you follow my advice you may meet with a bit of resistance. For example, in several states your right to a copy of your medical records is guaranteed by law, but you may still have difficulty in exercising your right. This guide outlines the likely obstacles you will face, and explains how to deal with those obstacles.

Some of these claims may seem a bit grandiose. But I assure you they are not. I have no inside knowledge or inside track yet I did most of the things that I advocate here. While it takes a bit of time and legwork it is not difficult to improve your prospects by empowering yourself through information.

I want to make clear that this guide is not meant to be an indictment of doctors. My feeling is that many of the criticisms lodged at physicians result from the expectations that we as patients have for those who are advising and treating us. Too often we expect them to have all the answers and solutions. We demand not only technical expertise in medicine, but also flawless interpersonal and communications skills, a sophisticated understanding of psychology, unlimited availability, and a potpourri of superhuman abilities. Sometimes, when doctors behave in ways that we consider arrogant, they are merely reflecting the image that patients have demanded they fulfill.

I also want to make clear that this guide does not advocate so-called alternatives, like foreign treatments of dubious scientific merit, cure by miracle diet, or cure by positive thinking. Indeed, I was treated and apparently cured by traditionally trained physicians with the skill to administer the latest drugs that were developed by traditional medical research. I just found out who those doctors were, what they were using, and how to get access to the treatment they were administering. ❖

❖

CHAPTER TWO

Finding Basic Information

C ancer is complex, even to scientists who have dedicated their careers to its study. You will not be able to learn all the intricate details of your illness, but you can learn the basics. In fact, within a day or so of your diagnosis you can learn a great deal about the illness you face and the treatment possibilities available to fight it.

This section covers some of the initial information gathering steps that will give you a basic understanding of your illness. Chapter eight outlines some more involved research steps that you can take to learn more about your illness and treatment options. I divided the two information gathering sections this way because I feel it makes sense chronologically. While basic information gathering is essential right after your diagnosis, other steps such as getting a second opinion and asking your doctor the right questions come before searching for more detailed information.

Neither this section nor the later one on information gathering is meant to be an exhaustive guide to cancer research. It is intended for the patient without medical research training, who wants to quickly gain a level of understanding of his disease and care options so he can participate in making informed care choices.

National Cancer Institute (NCI)

The National Cancer Institute is a U.S. government agency falling under the jurisdiction of the National Institute of Health. The NCI is one of the best single source of information for the cancer patient. Beside spending nearly 2 billion dollars per year on research, NCI also publishes booklets and pamphlets on cancer, maintains an 800 number telephone information and assistance line, and maintains Physician's Data Query (PDQ) an on-line computer database that makes the latest cancer information available to practitioners, researchers, and patients. The easiest way to access the NCI's formidable information resources is through their 800 number.

1-800-4-CANCER (1-800-422-6237)

Calling this phone number will put you in touch with the NCI's Cancer Information Service. NCI information specialists can answer some of your questions about cancer in general and about the specific kind of cancer that afflicts you. Be sure to ask about:

The PDQ Summary of Your Illness

The PDQ database contains summaries of the latest information on most types of cancer. It includes information on symptoms, diagnosis criteria, normal course of illness, staging, state of the art treatments, and treatments in clinical trial. The NCI Cancer Information Service staff people will read and explain the information to you in summary form and will send you a printout upon request. If there are clinical trials in progress the NCI can also send you the details including the location of the trial, the name of the lead researchers, and technical information including the phase of the trial. For more information on clinical trials, see chapter seven.

As far as I'm concerned every physician should be required to consult PDQ when making a cancer diagnosis. Such a requirement can help assure that patients are getting information about the latest treatments. In the absence of such a regulation, you will have to take responsibility for getting the PDQ report yourself.

It will take a few days to get the PDQ report from NCI, which may or may not be a problem for you. Another shortcoming of obtaining the PDQ report from NCI is that you will get only part of the full text as it relates to your illness. Although PDQ includes several sections on each illness, some of those sections are designed for patients while other sections are designed for practitioners. The Cancer Information Service people prefer to limit the amount of practitioner information sent to patients.

Accessing PDQ Directly
Anyone can easily access PDQ by subscribing to one of three on-line computer services—CompuServe, Dialog, or Medlars. If you have a

computer, a modem, communications software, and a credit card, you can subscribe to CompuServe, access PDQ, and have the report within minutes. Some sections of PDQ can be accessed directly via any fax machine. Chapter eight explains how you can sign up for CompuServe, and access PDQ directly through CompuServe and through other methods.

NCI Booklets

The NCI publishes and distributes, without charge, nearly 100 booklets and pamphlets about cancer. Ask the information specialist (through the 1-800-4-CANCER phone service) for any booklets that might be helpful to you specifically. A listing for the various NCI titles appears in appendix III. Two NCI series deserve mention here:

What You Need To Know About Cancer (series)

There are at least 26 booklets in this series, each dealing with a specific type of cancer. Each booklet offer a brief explanation of the kind of cancer with which it deals. In simple terms, each explains the illness, its symptoms, treatment, questions to ask your doctor, and includes a glossary of the terms with which you will want to become familiar.

Research Report (series)

This series includes more detailed reports on at least 18 specific kinds of cancer. Although these reports are a bit more technical and sophisticated than the *What You Need To Know About Cancer* series, they are generally well written and understandable to the lay person.

The research reports are aimed more at those who want to be informed participants in their own care. For example, the *What You Need To Know About Cancer* series starts its section on treatment with "Your doctor will consider a number of factors in determining the best treatment for you." The *Research Report* series explains the various treatment options including recent developments and directions, and a bibliography of relevant articles from medical journals. It does not remove the patient from the decision making process like the former series does.

The only problem with this series is the frequency of updating. I just received the Research Report on leukemia from the NCI. It was last revised over four years ago, an eternity in the world of cancer research. It discusses as being in clinical trial, a treatment for hairy cell leukemia that was approved by the FDA a year ago. The treatment that I received over a year ago is not even mentioned. Nevertheless, this series offers a good basis for understanding your illness, options, and prospects.

Getting NCI Information Quickly

According to one of the Cancer Information Service staffers I talked to, most direct patient requests for preprinted information (booklets) are sent within 24 hours by first class mail. PDQ information may take a few days to arrive. The information specialists will, at their discretion, rush certain requested items but they will not fax or send anything by overnight mail.

There are a couple options if you can't wait the few days that your request for information will take to fulfill.

Federal Depository Libraries

Many major U.S. libraries are designated as Federal Depository Libraries. They get government materials, such as NCI literature, directly from the government printing office and from government agencies. Not all designated libraries get all government literature, but they all get a good amount of it. The reference librarian at the main branch of your local library should be able to tell you if they are an FDL or, if not, where the nearest FDL is located. Most FDL's have trained staff available to help you locate the specific material that you are looking for.

Every Federal Depository Library is required to grant public access to the government document section of the library without charge or unreasonable restriction. If access to the library itself is restricted, merely explain that you are there to review government materials; you will be allowed in.

Visit An NCI Cancer Information Service Office

Although the CIS is designed primarily as a phone in service, all of its offices are open to the public. By visiting your regional office, you can probably leave with all the booklets that you need. You may even be able to persuade the staff to search PDQ for you while you are right there, and take the printout with you. The CIS people were reluctant to give me a full list of addresses of their offices. However, you can call the 1-800-4-CANCER number and ask the information specialist where the nearest office to you is located.

Cancer and Health Associations

Most people have heard of the larger private associations and societies that help fight cancer such as the American Cancer Society and the Leukemia Society of America. Besides these two giants, there are dozens of other private nonprofit groups dedicated to cancer research, information, and patient support. A listing and brief description of several of these organizations appears in appendix IV.

While the groups vary in their missions a call to those that specialize in your type of cancer is well worth the effort. Merely explain your situation and ask what kind of help they might offer. The Leukemia Society of America's local chapter alerted me to the fact that there was a new treatment in clinical trial for the kind of leukemia I had, and explained their policy of offering partial reimbursement of treatment related travel expenses for leukemia patients.

The American Cancer Society, the best known of the groups, recently announced that it plans to change its focus from cancer treatment to cancer prevention. ACS still maintains an 800 number for call-in help to patients and their families. It also still distributes free booklets on specific types of cancer. The ACS booklets seem to be quite basic with a lot of emphasis on statistics such as the number of people with the specific illness, survival rates, etc.

My own view is that the NCI publications are more useful than the ACS material. The ACS 800 call-in service too (1-800 ACS-2345) is decidedly less helpful than the NCI's call in service. It is staffed by volunteers who can arrange to send booklets and assist with local resources. They are not set-up to search the PDQ, or any other database.

A foundation that deserves special note is called the R.A. Bloch Cancer Support Center. This foundation, founded by Richard Bloch who also co-founded H&R Block, Inc. will provide second opinions to qualifying cancer patients. These second opinions are provided free of charge by a team of physicians from different medical specialties. See chapter six on the importance of getting a qualified second opinion. See appendix IV for the address and phone number of this organization.

Finally, it is sometimes worthwhile to also call an association that does not specialize in cancer, but in the organ where your cancer is located. For example if you suffer from thyroid cancer, call the American Thyroid Association or if you suffer from liver cancer call the American Liver Foundation. You can find associations dedicated to the health of several different human organs in the *Encyclopedia of Associations* (see appendix V).

Medical Textbooks

It could be helpful to you to buy a medical text that deals with your type of illness. Expect a text to have technical language and to assume knowledge beyond that of a lay person. Nevertheless, a text can serve as a reference to you that can be called upon to help you understand different aspects of your problem as you learn more about it.

The place to find medical textbooks is at medical school bookstores and other large bookstores with medical text departments. Browse through the different books on the specific medical area that you need to know about. Choose a text which you can at least partially understand and that seems to have a lot of information on your specific disease.

Unfortunately, medical texts will not necessarily have the latest information because new research reported since the time the book was printed can't be included. By the time the book is in the store, a year or more could have passed since it went to press. Also, be warned that medical texts are not cheap.

Three oncology textbooks that are used extensively are *Cancer Principles and Practice of Oncology* by Vincent T. DeVita, Jr., MD, et al., *Manual of Oncologic Therapeutics* edited by Robert E. Wittes, MD, and *Comprehensive Textbook of Oncology*, by A.R. Moossa, et al. See the bibliography for complete references (appendix V). ❖

CHAPTER THREE

❖

Evaluating Your Doctor

M ost of us evaluate doctors primarily based upon how nice they are. While a doctor's bedside manner and charisma are fine factors to consider, his technical competence and ability to communicate complex medical information to patients are more important considerations. Unfortunately, it is not easy for non-physicians to objectively judge a physician's technical competence. However, there are a few independent sources you can check to get some idea of your doctor's credentials and indications of previous malpractice or wrongdoing.

Directory of Medical Specialties — This reference guide provides information about virtually all licensed physicians practicing in the U.S.. Arranged by specialty, this guide includes information on each doctor's schooling and residency, affiliations, honors, and other information. While it contains the basics on just about every physician, the information is based on the physician's own reporting. Some physicians want every accolade listed while others do not so they don't point them out to the publisher. This guide is available at major public libraries, hospital libraries, and other libraries. See appendix V for bibliographic information.

State Licensing Boards — Practicing physicians, other than those working exclusively for the military or the federal government, must be licensed by the state(s) in which they practice. The various state licensing boards have somewhat different policies about providing information about a physician to the public. Most will confirm that a doctor is or is not in good standing with the licensing board. Most will also let you know if any type of disciplinary action was taken against a licensed physician by the board. Although a call to the state licensing board probably won't turn up much, it's worth a check. Look under your state's department of health listings in the telephone book.

Questionable Doctors — This publication lists medical doctors who have been censured or disciplined by a state licensing board. It also explains the reason for the disciplinary action. While you can get information on disciplinary action on a particular doctor through your state licensing board (see subsection above), this guide lists each doctor so you can easily check for a group of physicians.

It is available on a state by state basis at a price of $12.00 for the first state requested, and $5.00 for each additional state requested. See the bibliography (appendix V) for further ordering details

The Medical Community — The reference guides above are only of limited value in choosing a doctor. They are probably more helpful in eliminating a poor choice than in finding a good choice. If you have friends who are physicians, nurses, or other medical professionals, they may have insider knowledge on who is good, mediocre, and less than competent. Equally as important, people on the inside are in a good position to find out which doctors are especially knowledgeable in your particular type of cancer. Chapter six contains some additional information on finding doctors who are expert in your particular cancer. ❖

CHAPTER FOUR

❖

Questions to Ask Your Doctor

While this guide details several sources of information, your doctor is your first source. To get the information you need from your doctor, you need to ask the right questions. It is not fair to expect the doctor to know what questions you want answered unless you ask them. Some suggested questions are noted and explained below. It is not a complete list by any means. Different patients have different concerns. Before your next appointment, write down all the questions you have. Don't be afraid to ask questions that seem silly, stupid, or embarrassing. Most doctors are very accustomed to a wide range of patient concerns and questions. They will not be easily shocked by your questions. Even the worst case scenario of embarrassing yourself is well worth the information that you will get. The biggest fears of so many patients are in fact baseless supposition. Many fears could be alleviated if you can muster the courage to ask your doctor.

Some patients like to keep a notebook with them at all times so they can jot down questions as they think of them. You might want to tape record your question and answer session. Invariably people forget some of what was said at any meeting and reconstruct the contents in their mind. Especially in stressful situations, we all tend to hear what we want to hear to some degree or utilize what psychologists call selective perception. If not a tape recorder, at least bring a notebook and take notes.

Many patients like to bring someone else with them to the meeting where details of their condition will be explained. Under the difficult circumstances, a spouse, friend, or relative may be helpful in processing, taking notes on, and remembering what the doctor has said, and in asking appropriate questions.

Finally, be sure to get the correct spelling for technical terms such as the full name of your illness, the full name of any drugs or other treatments proposed, of any tests you're asked to take, potential side effects, and potential complications. Without the full name and spelling, your research efforts will be hampered.

Suggested Questions-Illness and Treatment

Exactly what do I have?
If you plan to research your condition, it is not enough to know that you have breast cancer, leukemia, or skin cancer. Most categories of cancer have a number of variations, all with different specific names, prognoses, and treatment options.

At what stage is the disease?
The kind of cancer you have and the point to which it has progressed, determine how much time you can wait before you get treatment. Some cancers are clearly staged in steps such as 1-5. Other are measured by size, by cell appearance, or by other indicators such as blood counts or blood chemistry. Knowing the stage and the signs of progression will enable you to track your illness along with your doctor. It can also help in examining various treatments options because different treatments are better suited to different stages.

What is the normal progression of this disease?
Physicians are understandably reluctant to make specific predictions about how long terminally ill patients have to live. Nevertheless, you need to know what will likely happen as the disease progresses. The answer to this question will help you make a number of decisions, and give you an idea of the time pressures that you may face. Insist on a straight answer, even if the answer is not what you want to hear.

It might be beneficial to ask the physician to explain the range of possibilities rather than its normal course. This wording might make the doctor less uncomfortable, and his response more complete and honest. It also may give you more useful information.

What are the markers for progression or improvement of disease?
The progression of most kinds of cancers is charted by tests and symptoms known as markers. The spread of some types of lymphomas, for example, are charted by the number of lymph nodes where cancerous cells are found, and by the presence or absence of

fever. While you may not immediately understand the indicators or markers, a little background study will bring you up to speed on the basics.

What are current treatment options?
What are the pros and cons of each?
What are the short and long term side effects of each?
These questions will not only provide the information you need toward making your decisions, it will also test your physician's knowledge of the treatment alternatives. Crisp direct answers indicate he is versed in the treatment possibilities. Vague or overly simplistic answers or reluctance to answer indicates either that the doctor is not versed in treatment of your illness or that he does not think that patients should have this vital information.

The answers themselves will give you a clearer idea of the kinds of decisions you face and your prospects with each choice.

What is the goal of treatment?
In some cases the goal is to manage or palliate the illness. In other cases it is to induce a remission (a lessening of the disease for a period of time). Sometimes the goal is outright cure—complete eradication of the disease.

Are there any treatments in clinical trial?
Clinical trials are at the cutting edge in combating cancer. If there are clinical trials in progress for your particular kind of cancer, you will want to know about them.

Your doctor may not know the answer to this question. If he does, it indicates that he is up-to-date on the latest information available. If he offers to find out for you, it indicates that he is open to new developments.

You might get disapproval from the physician for this line of questioning. For example, some physicians equate clinical trials with human guinea pig experimentation. Don't be deterred. The risks vary and you can and will get more information before proceeding with or deciding against a clinical trial. Far more people are helped than hurt by clinical trials. My own treatment was a clinical trial. Former U.S. Senator and presidential candidate Paul Tsongas' long remission was induced through a clinical trial. Clinical trials are covered in more detail in chapter seven.

Do you tend to be aggressive, conservative, or in the middle?
Doctors vary as to their degree of preferred risk taking when it comes to treating cancer. Some prefer to intervene as little as possible, others are anxious to use the most potent cancer weapons available, while some take a middle of the road stand. You should think about your own feelings regarding an aggressive versus a conservative approach and understand your physician's position so you can decide how well his inclinations match your own.

What do you recommend at this point?
You will certainly want to know your own doctor's treatment proposal and the reasons for his recommendations.

Are there other treatment choices of which you are aware?
Once you know the various options, it is up to you to choose the option that you like best. It is not unusual at all for a disease to have two, three, or more treatment protocols. Don't assume that your doctor's recommendation is the only choice or even the best choice for you.

What are the risks and expected side effects of the various options?
Unfortunately, when you have cancer you have to make decisions that involve significant risk. Many treatments involve powerful drugs—essentially poisons that can destroy cancer cells but also damage healthy cells in the process. Other treatments involve potentially dangerous surgery or radiation. You may be faced with the choice of accepting more risk for the chance of more complete remission or even cure. In some instances the risks are well understood. In other situations, such as clinical trials, all the possible long term side effects and risk are not always known.

What would you do in my situation?
This questions looks like the previous one but when asked this way, the response may be very different. In my experience, it seems to make the doctor stop and think in more personal and human terms. An honest answer to this question carries a good deal of weight.

How will my life be impaired now?
How will it be impaired after treatment?
If you will be living with handicaps, you need to know what they are

so you can prepare to deal with them. Also, the handicaps and side effects of different alternatives are an important factor in making your treatment choices.

What precautions should I take?
When I got my diagnosis of leukemia my white blood count was quite low leaving me especially vulnerable to infectious illness. Further, if I caught an infectious illness, my immune system would have had a difficult time fighting it off. However, the doctor did not tell me this until I asked him directly if I were especially vulnerable to infectious illness. He answered, yes, and wrote a prescription for an antibiotic to be taken if and when I did get sick.

A man I know with the same diagnosis as I was told to take aspirin for an unrelated problem by a doctor treating him for that unrelated problem. He then developed three bleeding ulcers. His leukemia left him with low platelets and aspirin is known to decrease the effectiveness of platelets. The ulcers may not have occurred had his platelets been normal. The aspirin then may well have contributed to his ulcers. Had he asked his oncologist about precautions and restrictions, the bleeding ulcers might have been avoided.

It is important to make other health care providers aware of your condition and the necessary precautions. For example, three months after my diagnosis, I developed a toothache. My dentist prescribed a root canal which I agreed to after telling him that I had hairy cell leukemia. I naively assumed that he would know if my condition might be a factor to consider before proceeding. This incident became one of my early lessons in ceding responsibility for health care decisions. The root canal became infected and other complications developed. The day after the infection surfaced was also the day of my second opinion. I mentioned the problem to the oncologist who examined me. She admonished me for allowing the dentist to perform an invasive procedure and insisted that I have no more such procedures. She then called the dentist and the two of them worked out a strategy to undo the damage that should not have been done in the first place.

Is there a chance of central nervous system involvement?
For me it was easier to ask if I was about to die than if the disease would somehow destroy or impair my mind. But I had to know the

answer so I could make whatever plans I had to make. Fortunately, the answer in my case was no as it is with most kinds of cancer. Of course you will want to know if any treatment being considered can affect your own brain functioning.

How much do you know about this particular illness?
Is there another doctor with whom I should consult?
You want to establish the degree of expertise and experience your doctor has in your particular illness. You can soft peddle the question if it will make it easier for you (How many others with this illness have you treated?, Is this your specialty?, etc.) but get the answer. You are paying the doctor for his expertise. If he lacks expertise in the area where you most need it, find another doctor. Again, concern about preserving your life should take precedent over worrying about protecting your doctor's feelings.

Will you work with other experts in my treatment?
It is not unusual for practicing physicians to seek the advice and guidance of other physicians at major research centers. For example, physicians at research centers may prescribe protocols and dosages, while the local practitioner actually administers the treatment and follows the patient's progress. Ask your doctor if he ordinarily enters into this type of relationship. A doctor who is closed to this possibility is a doctor to be avoided.

How much will treatment (and pre and post treatment observation and follow up) cost?
How much of it will insurance cover?
Doctors don't always like to discuss the money aspects of care and treatment with patients, but you need to know the answers. If cost is a factor for you, you need to make appropriate arrangements. It may be as easy as switching from a physician who does not participate in your health plan to one that does. It may unfortunately be far more complex than that too, but you need to know what you are up against.

Many doctors, especially those on hospital staffs full time, do not know about the financial aspects of treatment. If the doctor does not know the answers to the financial questions or is reluctant to answer, he should be able to tell you where to find the information that you need.

Questions Regarding Tests

Modern medicine is blessed with many types of diagnostic tests, including some high technology tests that were unimaginable just a few years ago. These tests are very helpful in diagnosing, planning treatment, and measuring the progress of illness or treatment. However, not every test ordered by a physician is essential. There is a range; some tests are crucial, some helpful, and some marginal. Don't hesitate to ask the ordering physician about the tests' purpose, relative importance, and about any risks to you from the tests. You may elect to pass on a long and painful test to eliminate a one in two-thousand possibility as a factor in your illness. Then again, you may be reassured by having every possibility explored.

The fear of malpractice suits has created a situation where doctors will sometimes order tests more for legal than medical reasons. There are cases where a doctor will be convinced based upon his own professional judgment, that a certain diagnosis is highly unlikely. However, he also understands that juries are not as impressed by professional judgment as they are by laboratory and other high tech testing procedures. The fear of a malpractice suit will thus make doctors err on the side of caution— even over-caution— and order superfluous tests as part of the practice of defensive medicine.

Even if you elect to proceed with every test the doctor requests, it is psychologically helpful to understand the benefits of those tests. Some patients, who have no idea why they are having a series of tests done report feeling like human guinea pigs.

The Patient's Guide to Medical Tests, by Cathey and Edward Pinckney, describes a number of medical tests including how they work, their risks, and their accuracy. It also contains some good information on medical testing in general. See appendix V for bibliographic information.

These questions are only a few of the basics. You should think about all your questions in advance, write them down, and bring them with you to your appointments. Most doctors will be happy to answer your questions. If yours is not, find one who is.

However, the doctor will not be able to spend a great deal of time with you; he has other patients who need his expertise too. That is one reason that you should not consider this brief question and answer session your only chance to learn about your illness and your options. This is the first step. The rest of this guide covers other sources for finding background information as well as the latest technical information. ❖

❖

CHAPTER FIVE

Your Medical Records

Your medical records document your medical history, tests, diagnoses, physician recommendations, treatments, and related details. They are essential to the management of your illness. Most patient's records are never seen by the patient whose medical life they document. Despite the fact that access to your records is often guaranteed by law, many physicians and health care personnel discourage patient access to those records. Regardless of your doctor's feelings on releasing your records to you, getting your records is an essential step in your search for information.

Why You Need Your Records

Obtaining your current medical records is important for a number of reasons:

a. General Research — To find out about your condition, you need to know what that condition is. The name of your illness is not sufficient. Details about your diagnosis, such as its stage and its progress, impact upon your prospects and your options. Those details are not found in the name of your illness, but are found in your records.

b. Asking Questions — The more you know, the more you realize how much you don't know. Studying your records will foster many questions about your condition. Asking your doctor for explanations will further your understanding of your situation.

c. Second Opinion — The next section of this booklet discusses the need for a second opinion. The doctor you see for your second opinion will probably insist that you bring your records with you. Even if he does not insist on it, having those records available can only help you to get more value from that second opinion. Don't depend on a promise by the hospital or doctor's office to forward your records directly to the new doctor. The only way to be sure the records will be there is if you take responsibility for their delivery.

d. Treatment — If you opt to be treated by a physician other than your current doctor, the treating doctor will need your records. Don't assume that the system works so well that your records will reach the treating doctor merely because you requested that they be sent. If you don't take responsibility to get them to the treating doctor, they may be delayed, and your treatment may be delayed because of it.

e. Monitoring — Biological changes need to be closely monitored to chart the progress of most cancers. For example, blood counts for leukemia patients provide an indicator as to the progress of the disease.

Passive patients assume that their doctor is on top of every laboratory test, X-ray, and related test. In reality, a busy doctor can easily miss an essential indicator or marker. If you learn what the markers are, you can then watch closely for them and be sure that your physician is made aware of a development that might be important.

f. Tracking Progress — If you are undergoing periodic testing, you can chart your own progress as long as you have access to the information. If all is going well, you will know it and be more at ease because of it. If there are signs of concern, you will be able to make sure that you get attention quickly.

Where Your Records Are

Hospitals and large clinics have whole departments that maintain patient records. These departments are called, logically enough, medical records departments. Patient records are stored in these departments unless they are checked out to an authorized physician. In the more high tech institutions, some parts of the patient records are stored on computer and can be electronically examined by a physician without physically leaving the medical records department's computers.

Private practice physicians also keep detailed patient records. Only the largest practices have separate medical records departments, but all have the records and typically have someone who is in charge of maintaining those records.

Access to Your Records

In this country today, citizens are guaranteed access to much of what is recorded about us. Federal law guarantees, for example, access to one's own credit file held by credit bureaus. Even copies of any records held by the FBI or CIA are accessible to us through the Freedom of Information Act. Despite the objections of educators, our school records too are available to us upon request. However, in many states, there are no laws guaranteeing a patient access to his medical records.

Many individuals and organizations are working to change this archaic form of censorship. In fact, considerable headway has been made in recent years in that 26 states currently have adopted laws making the release of records to patients mandatory in nearly all instances, and other states have laws making records partially available.

Even the American Medical Association, which once stood against patient access to records, has changed its policy to one that encourages doctors to provide patients with copies of records upon written request.

Further, most accredited hospitals subscribe to a set of principles formulated by the American Hospital Association, known as the Patient Bill of Rights. One of those rights is your right to review your records.

Legalities

The law differs from state to state. Some states insist upon full patient access records. Other states have laws demanding that hospitals make records available to patients, but have no such requirement for private practice physicians. At least one state has the reverse: private practice physicians must make records available to the patient, but hospitals are not forced to do the same.

Some state laws make release of records mandatory only if good cause is demonstrated by the patient.

No state currently has laws that specifically prohibit patient access to records. However, in the absence of a law pertaining to access to records, a patient may be denied such access.

Federally operated medical facilities, such as Veterans Administration hospitals, are governed by federal law instead of state law. Under the Federal Privacy Act, a patient's records held by U.S. government facilities are accessible to that patient.

In many instances where access to records is guaranteed by law, the patient must make a formal written request to the hospital or the private practice physician asking that the records to be released.

The easiest way to find out your own state's current laws pertaining to this issue is to call your state's department of health, physician licensing board, or your own attorney.

You may also call or write the People's Medical Society in Allentown PA (see appendix IV for phone number and address). They will tell you the law in your state and, provide you with a sample letter that can be used to request your records.

Obtaining Your Records

Clearly, if you (or more specifically your records) are in a state that guarantees patient access to records, you are in a better position than if you are in a state without such enlightened regulations. Nevertheless, you may well encounter obstacles to exercising your legal rights.

Regardless of the law, the medical system resists handing records over to patients. It's hard to imagine the kind of sinister use the powers that be think patients will find for their records but obstacles are sometimes constructed to keep you and your records apart. Perhaps they understand that the patient with his own records has power that they would rather see reserved for their own hands.

For example, I once obtained my records from a private practice physician and from a hospital. I went to a new doctor at a different hospital, records in hand. The doctor asked if he could keep a copy; I agreed. His secretary took the records to copy. I made the mistake of leaving without remembering to bring the records with me.

Scripps Clinic, the clinic that ultimately treated me, called asking that I send my complete records to them as soon as possible. I called the doctor and explained my oversight and the Scripps request. He said he was on his way out of town but would leave a note with the medical records department explaining that I would be picking up my records.

The medical records people gave me lots of forms to fill out and said they would call when the records were ready (I'm not sure what getting them ready entailed. Maybe they had to clean them off or check for neatness). A day went by with no call, so I called them, politely asking for my records again. They explained that they could not give them to me. I figured I could clear things up by pointing out that both Rhode Island law and the patient bill of rights to which the hospital subscribed guaranteed my access to these records. Boy was I naive!

The clerk, probably after categorizing and labeling me a difficult patient, put me in touch with the supervisor who explained that they could not release records from a private practice physician nor from another hospital. She was not impressed with the fact that I physically brought those records to the hospital, nor my argument that I, not the hospital, owned these copies of my records, nor my doctor's written note asking that the records be given to me. She was no more impressed by my logic that since the other hospital and the private practice doctor were all in Rhode Island, the law would prohibit them from denying access to my records.

It got straightened out several days and several threats later, but this dispute delayed my treatment unnecessarily.

The medical records people in this situation argued, with some legal justification, that they were not permitted to release records from another institution. At best however, my case falls into a gray area in that the records were not forwarded to them by another institution but were given to them by me. There are three lessons to take from this story. First, gray area decisions regarding patient records tend to be decided against releasing those records to the patient. Second, get your records from each hospital or physician's office directly. Do not assume you can wait until your records are all together in one place and you can save yourself several steps by picking them up as a complete package. Finally, once you have your records in hand, do not give them up without making at least one full set of copies.

Stories like mine are common, even in states where the laws are with the patient. Even in states that don't guarantee access, assertive and persistent patients will usually prevail and get their records. When they do, those handing over the records will often make a pathetic attempt at maintaining their perceived power by sealing them in an envelope that says something like "For Doctor John Doe only."

If You Have Problems Getting Your Records

Those in the medical establishment know that most patients will never request a copy of their records for their own use. Even most of those who do, will not be aware of their legal rights and will, more often than not, back down. So you're up against not only the system's reluctance to cooperate, but also its security in knowing that it can usually get away without cooperating.

Once you prove you will not back down, you should be able to get what you're after. If you do run into difficulty in getting your records, remain cool but assertive. Remember that your request is legitimate and those resisting it will eventually comply if you keep up your insistence.

Make your request in writing. AMA policy and some state laws insist upon a written request by the patient. Don't get carried away in explaining why you want the records unless the law requires that you show cause or state your need for the records.

If your state has no access laws and your request is rejected or ignored, a call to your lawyer may be in order. Also, as mentioned above, the People's Medical Society in Allentown, Pennsylvania can advise you as to the current law in your state as it pertains to patient access to records. They will also send you a sample letter that can be used to request your records.

Finally, it may be easier to persuade those who are blocking access to your records to send them directly to another doctor or hospital. This procedure is more traditional so it is less likely to meet with strident resistance. It is degrading to have to resort to this method that treats you like a child, but it you are less concerned with taking a stand and more concerned with efficiently dealing with your health problems, it may be the path to take.

29

Examining Your Records

While it is essential that you get your records, it is not essential that you fully understand them; in all likelihood, you will not. You need them to get your second opinion (see next section) and to start your information gathering. However, they are your starting point for your research, not your end point. From your records, you will learn what you need to learn about.

Doctors sometimes make notes within the records of a number of possible diagnoses. Don't be frightened by this. It does not mean that you have or are likely to have any of the conditions mentioned in note form. Such notes merely indicate that your doctor is (or was) considering these possibilities. Pay more attention to pathology reports and formal statements by your physician that diagnose your condition.

A good medical dictionary will be helpful in interpreting your records. Finally, make sure you get clarification on points you don't understand either from the diagnosing physician, or the physician who you see for your second opinion. ❖

CHAPTER SIX

❖

Getting a Second Opinion

A gentleman in Florida whom I'll call Frank was in his early sixties when he was diagnosed with a form of liver cancer about four years ago. His doctor told him that nothing could be done for him; he had only months to live. His brother-in-law, a hospital administrator, insisted he immediately get a second opinion from a major cancer research center. Frank decided it would be a waste of time because his doctor, who he trusted completely, was quite clear on his prognosis.

Frank's brother-in-law was adamant. As the story was told to me he made an appointment for Frank at the Mayo Clinic and, despite Frank's protests and skepticism, practically forced him to get on the plane to Minnesota.

I don't know if Frank ever said thank you to his despotic brother-in-law but I know he should have. You see, the doctors at Mayo operated on Frank quite successfully. Their parting words to him were, "we don't expect to see you back here with this problem." So far the Mayo physicians expectations have been fulfilled. Frank has not needed any more cancer treatment from the Mayo doctors or from any doctors for that matter. He is alive and doing well today. His continued life is a vivid illustration of the value of the second opinion.

Medicine, especially as it applies to the complexities of cancer, is not an exact science. It is not unusual for two doctors, faced with the same data, to put forth two different opinions as to diagnoses and treatment. It is no less unusual for one's doctor to not have all the latest information on the illness for which he is proposing treatment.

Unless a delay of a few days would be life threatening, a second opinion is essential. The second opinion is a centerpiece of insuring that you are aware of the alternatives and that the proposed treatment is the best option for you.

If you decide to follow only one piece of advice in this booklet, follow this one: *Get a second opinion from a physician well versed in your disease and its treatment options.*

Surprisingly, many patients just don't do this. Few people would buy the first house, car, or major appliance they see without checking to see what other options might be available. Yet when it comes to the infinitely higher stakes choice—which path to take in one's attempt to survive—so many people find a dozen justifications to take the easy path and forego the second opinion.

Why the Reluctance to Get a Second Opinion?

Why are the same people who insist on say, test driving several cars before choosing one, reluctant to get a second opinion when it comes to saving their life? I've asked patients and doctors this question. The most common answer seems to be that patients fear offending their doctor.

In the early phases of my own cancer story I was advised by two doctors that I knew socially to get a second opinion. Both explained that I would need to obtain my medical records from the diagnosing doctor first. Both also advised me on how I should gingerly explain my decision to get another opinion to my doctor, even suggesting helpful white lies. I was a bit puzzled as to why the approach was so important to them. They certainly knew that in Rhode Island patients are guaranteed access to their medical records so persuading the doctor to relinquish them to me was not an issue.

Later I called the internist who referred me to my initial oncologist partly to ask if he had a recommendation as to who I should see for a second opinion. He too suggested how I might gently approach the subject with Dr. Telder. However, midway through his advice on diplomacy, he stopped and said "Well I guess protecting your doctor's feelings is not the most important thing to you right now." Bingo! What I didn't say but felt was "I don't want to be insensitive but if the search for a better chance at surviving means I might have to risk hurting my doctor's feelings a bit, well, that's a small price to pay."

In all likelihood your insistence on getting another opinion will not be too much of a bruise to your doctor's ego. Most physicians, especially those involved in the complexities of cancer care, are accustomed to the fact that some patients seek second opinions. Physician's themselves, when faced with a serious illness, invariably seek multiple opinions. If your doctor is insulted by your request, well that's too bad. He'll get over it.

Why A Second Opinion is Necessary

A Physician Can't be Up-to-Date on Every Development.
Medicine is very much a high technology field. As with any high tech field, evolutionary and revolutionary developments are constantly surfacing. It is not fair to expect any practitioner to be up to date on every current development. Eight years ago the most current treatment available for my kind of leukemia was splenectomy. Six years ago the then new drug, interferon-alpha was approved by the FDA for the treatment of hairy cell leukemia. Following on its heels was a drug called 2-deoxycoformycin which was in clinical trial at the time, and was ultimately approved by the FDA in 1991. In 1991 also, 2-CDA, the drug that seems to have saved me, was well into clinical trial. By 1992, 2-CDA was designated as a group C investigational drug by the National Cancer Institute meaning that the FDA had authorized NCI to distribute it to oncologists on a request basis because it had been so successful in trial. This drug will probably be fully approved for commercialization by the FDA this year (1993) and will probably antiquate the previous three treatments, two of which were not even available eight years ago.

A doctor who is busy practicing medicine just doesn't have time to closely watch the ever changing field of medical research on behalf of every patient. An article in the March 1992 issue of *Consumer Reports* cites a study by sociologist David Phillips of the University of California at San Diego that found most physicians initially get their information on new medical developments from the newspaper. Only a few developments make it into the daily paper right away; many never do at all.

It is quite possible that there is a better treatment available or in development about which your doctor simply does not know. One possible way to find out if this is so in your case is simply to go to another doctor. See the section below *Where to Get a Second Opinion* (in chapter six) for information on the best places to go to for the latest opinion on treatment options, places where the doctors use information sources other than the daily newspaper.

Aggressive Doctors and Conservative Doctors

The possibility that a doctor lacks knowledge about a particular illness is not the only issue. Very competent specialists do not always agree on which treatment option is best. The same risk that one doctor might consider justified because of the possibility of a better outcome, another might shy away from reasoning that the risk is too great despite the possible but uncertain benefit. Both views are legitimate and defensible. What is inappropriate is for a doctor to force his or her bias on a patient who doesn't know that there are alternatives.

While some doctors will explain the options and explain their own personal bias on the conservative to aggressive spectrum, others will merely offer their treatment proposal as if it were the only reasonable option. A second opinion may give you a more or a less aggressive strategy to consider. You are the one who, armed with the facts on risk and benefits, should decide whether you want to be conservative or aggressive in your treatment.

Where to Get Your Second Opinion

The National Cancer Institute is the federal organization charged with the responsibility of coordinating government efforts toward fighting cancer. With its nearly two billion dollar annual budget, the NCI sponsors research and clinical trials, collects and distributes cancer information, and sponsors other programs and activities to battle cancer. Much of the research sponsored is carried out by other public and private organizations but with financial help from the NCI.

The NCI has designated twenty-eight hospitals and clinics as comprehensive cancer centers and twelve as clinical cancer centers. These centers have been recognized for their excellence in cancer treatment by the NCI. To be designated as a comprehensive cancer center, an institution must meet the following criteria:

-must pass rigorous peer review
-must have a strong core of basic laboratory research in several scientific fields
-must have a record of innovative clinical research studies
-must have a strong program of clinical research and an ability to transfer research findings into clinical practice
-must maintain strong participation in NCI designated high-priority clinical trials
-must maintain significant levels of cancer prevention and control research
-must initiate outreach and educational activities
-must maintain cancer information services for patients and health professionals

The clinical cancer centers focus on both basic research and clinical research within each institution. They frequently incorporate nearby affiliated clinical research institutions into their overall research programs.

If you possibly can, get a second opinion from a designated comprehensive cancer center. Failing that, a clinical cancer center would also be a good bet for a state of the art second opinion. The designated centers are required to keep up to date on the latest information about cancer and to participate in cancer research and clinical trials.

Also, their staffs include research physicians as well as full time practitioners. Research physicians tend to be up on the latest developments and the pros and cons of different treatment alternatives. Also, researchers at NCI designated facilities are more likely to seek out the latest information on a particular illness because they see that as part of their professional responsibility. Practitioners on the other hand, may tend to put a lower priority on keeping current with the latest research developments.

Appendix II. contains a listing of all the NCI comprehensive care centers and clinical care centers as of late 1992.

Finally, it is important to note that there are many other excellent cancer treatment facilities that do not have the NCI recognition as either a comprehensive or clinical cancer center. Other groups offer their own lists of quality cancer treatment institutions. For example, a magazine for cancer survivors and patients called *Coping*, publishes an annual listing of what it considers to be the top one-hundred institutions for cancer treatment in this country. See appendix V for information on this publication.

Getting an Appointment

Highly regarded physicians with cancer expertise seldom have an abundance of openings. However, they usually can make time available. While the traditional method of getting an appointment is by calling the hospital or the doctor's office and booking with a secretary, this may not be the best strategy. Despite the fact that your illness may have shaken your own world, your needs will not alter an institution's policies for setting up appointments. Medical support staffs deal with cancer patients regularly and become desensitized to their difficulties.

The physician himself, however, exercises at least some control over his own scheduling and can make decisions on squeezing patients in regardless of the length of his waiting list or the institution's policies. Getting priority for yourself might be possible if you know how to work the system.

Using Referrals

Like most professions, the medical profession favors its own. The vast majority of patients seen by cancer specialists have been referred by another doctor. If you call a cancer specialist yourself without a referral you are at a disadvantage. Some offices and hospitals have official policies of seeing patients by referral only. Others do not have such official policies but they nevertheless prefer to, and are accustomed to, filling a doctor's schedules this way.

Getting your own physician to call though is not always the most efficient strategy. For one thing, your doctor may be less than cooperative in assisting you in getting that second opinion or you may be uncomfortable in asking. For another, some doctors are more equal than others in the eyes of various specialists. While a referral by another doctor is better than no referral, a higher quality referral is better still. The hierarchy of referrals below is based on my own observations:

Referral Hierarchy

A Doctor Friend of the Doctor — If you are fortunate enough to have a friend who is a doctor, who is also a friend of the doctor that you want to see (we'll call the doctor you want to see your target doctor), you should have no difficulty getting an appointment quickly and easily. Merely prevail upon your friend to make an advance call for you and either set up an appointment or leave your name so when you call later, the office staff will find an appointment even if there are none available.

A Non MD Friend of the Doctor — If you know someone who plays golf or plays bridge with the doctor you want to see that person is certainly in a good position to ask for a favor on your behalf.

Well Known Physicians or Physicians With Brand Name Affiliation — Every field and subfield has its superstars. A referral that carries the name of a superstar physician, especially if that superstar is a cancer specialist, carries a great deal of weight. Even a doctor unknown to your chosen specialist, but with an affiliation such as an NCI designated comprehensive cancer facility or another highly regarded research site, is a quality referral.

At first blush, this seems like the hardest kind of referral to get. How can you get a well known doctor from a major research facility, to make a referral for you? Paradoxically, this can be one of the easiest kinds of referrals to gain because with a bit of maneuvering, legwork, and assertiveness, you can arrange for it yourself. Here's what to do:

Find out the names of three or four physicians in the field known as experts in your particular illness. You can do this at least three different ways:

a. Clinical Trial Lead Researchers — If you already know of a clinical trial involving your kind of cancer, find out who is leading it. For information on clinical trials including how to find out who is conducting clinical trials involving your illness, see chapters seven and eight.

b. Check professional articles and textbooks — If you research current journal articles and current textbooks in the field of your type of cancer, you'll see that the same names tend to be cited again and of cancer, you'll see that the same names tend to be cited again and again. Once you have the names and the affiliation (hospital, university, etc.) finding that doctor's address and phone number is relatively simple.

c. Ask your doctor — Your current doctor should know who in his field is making headlines through groundbreaking research. Even if the name you get is not that of the person who is doing the best and latest research, it is likely to be the name of a doctor who commands the respect of his peers.

The next step is to call one or more of the doctors whose names you obtained through one of these methods. Let's suppose the doctor that you learned about is conducting a clinical trial involving the cancer type that you have. Let's further pretend that his name is Dr. William Leader. You may not be able to speak directly with Dr. Leader, but that's OK. Explain to his secretary, nurse, or research assistant that you are interested in the experimental treatment he is running, and you would like to see him. If the doctor you are calling is not involved in a current trial merely explain that you know that he is a leading expert in the field of the cancer you have and that you would like his opinion.

Two things may happen. You may get an appointment, in which case you're all set. More likely, the assistant will explain that you need a referral from another doctor or for whatever reason, an appointment can not be set up so easily. In this case you explain that your current doctor is not familiar with Dr. Leader's work and not enthusiastic about assisting you in making a referral. Then ask if Dr. Leader would be so kind as to refer you to a doctor who might be more sympathetic to his treatment (or his work or diagnostic skills). Tell the assistant where you are located but also explain that you are willing to travel wherever necessary.

If Dr. Leader's office does not call you back within a day or two, don't be afraid to follow up with another call, and another until you get what you're after.

Once you get the name(s) you're after, call the doctor to whom Dr. Leader "referred" you. Now, armed with a referral from a leading physician in the field (Dr. Leader), you should have little difficulty getting an appointment. What's more, if you really are interested in

Dr. Leader's clinical trial and his own referral now turns around and refers you to him, you have a top quality entrée to get into the trial.

I did precisely as I advocate here. When I was considering the treatment that I ultimately received, there were two U.S. authorized clinical trial sites. I contacted both of them requesting a referral to a doctor familiar with the treatment and my own relatively rare disorder. I explained that I was in Rhode Island and that regional travel was not a problem; quality was most important. I ended up with two referrals in New York City (about 3 and a half hours by car). In both cases, the mention of my referral source got their immediate attention and easy access to their appointment books.

After receiving my second opinion from one of the two doctors, access to the clinical trial treatment that I wanted was all but assured. While the names of the doctors in New York meant nothing to me, a local doctor friend was more than a little impressed that I was so easily able to see the top people in his field.

A Doctor that the Doctor You Want to See Deals With Professionally

A doctor whom your target doctor sees regularly in the hospital hallway, at professional meetings or in other setting is a great referral source. Your target doctor knows that any lack of cooperation on his part might result in bad will on the part of his colleague. The fact that the two doctors see each other means that his cooperation or lack thereof will be recalled again and again every time their paths cross.

Your Current Primary Care Doctor

Typically, patients are referred to specialist by primary care physicians. You might well have first seen your internist who referred you to an oncologist or surgeon. It is neither unusual nor inappropriate for a patient to call the doctor who made the original referral and request another referral for a second opinion.

Additional Hints on Arranging
A Second Opinion

If You Know a Doctor Socially

As with most professions, practitioners extend professional courtesy to one another. That courtesy is often extended to friends of physicians. If your doctor friend calls your target doctor and asks him to see his friend, you then gain a level of status above that of an ordinary patient. This can not only get you the appointment your after, but may get it more quickly. Further, because that doctor knows you are likely to tell your friend how it went, he will be more careful in his examinations and recommendations.

Recently our family pediatrician took a new out-of-town job leaving us without a pediatrician. She gave us a short list of pediatricians whom she recommended. I called each one but was told that new patients were not being accepted at this time.

I told this to a doctor friend of mine who I'll call Sharon Jones. She asked the name of the pediatrician on the list that we thought would be best for us. Two days later Sharon called me. "That pediatrician you wanted. I spoke to him; you're all set. Call his office and tell the secretary you're a friend of Dr. Sharon Jones." I did. The next week both my kids were in his office.

Going Out of Town For Your Second Opinion

If you live in a relatively small community, you might want to get your second opinion outside of the immediate area. To some degree, physicians are reluctant to disagree with colleagues they know personally. In a small town where there are only a few practitioners of each sub-specialty, doctors see one another at local conferences, hospitals, or lectures. It can be a bit uncomfortable for a doctor to see and talk with the colleague whose opinion he recently discarded as inappropriate. ❖

CHAPTER SEVEN

❖

Clinical Trials and Medical Research

E very year in this country, billions of dollars are spent on research into cancer treatment. Much of this research takes place in laboratories utilizing test tubes and other scientific apparatus. Some experimentation takes place on animals. Only the most promising and safe anti-cancer agents and techniques are administered to humans. Cancer research projects involving human treatments are called clinical trials.

By nature, clinical trials are at the cutting edge of cancer treatments. It is here that the most promising developments are first tried and evaluated. Thousands of people, including myself, are alive and healthy today thanks to clinical trials. Virtually all anti-cancer drugs that are currently in use in this country (and in most other developed countries) are, or at one time were, in clinical trial. Virtually all anti-cancer drugs approved for use in this country were in clinical trials in this country regardless as to whether they were developed in foreign nations. The FDA insists on the submission of data from extensive U.S. trials before approving a drug.

But these trials are widely misunderstood in terms of risk, benefit, and availability. Many people, including some medical practitioners, frown upon clinical trials and denounce them as human guinea pig experimentation. While it is certainly fair to call clinical trials experiments, the potential benefits to the participating patient and to future cancer patients are undeniable.

Clinical trials that take place in this country must adhere to strict ethical standards and must be firmly based upon the principles of scientific inquiry. Much of the confusion about clinical trials comes about because those principles of scientific inquiry are not understood by many non-scientists. So before explaining the details of clinical trials, I'll overview the principles of scientific research.

Science Versus Supposition

Not long ago I was listening to the car radio on a long drive home. A gentleman was being interviewed on a talk show about how he cured himself of colon cancer. This gentleman claimed he refused all medical treatment and instead went on a macrobiotic diet which completely eradicated his cancer. Further, he was sure that most cancer sufferers could cure their disease through following his diet.

Was his cancer really cured through his macrobiotic diet? Maybe yes and maybe no. If his cancer really did disappear, there could have been any number of factors that independently or in combination with other factors were responsible for his reversal of fortune.

While it is entirely possible that the claimed disappearance of his cancer occurred concurrently with his macrobiotic diet, this in and of itself does not prove that his diet was the cause. Likewise, one person being treated with a drug and having his cancer disappear concurrently with that treatment does not prove the drug was the cause.

The key to proving or at least indicating a viable cause and effect relationship lies in the scientific method of inquiry. This first step of the scientific method involves isolating the substance or practice that is suspected of causing the outcome. That is isolating the variable — in this case the macrobiotic diet or the drug— from all other variables that might be alternative causes of the outcome. The scientific method also demands that results be duplicated several times before any reasonable cause and effect conclusions can be drawn.

Some phenomena are easy to prove scientifically. A healthy person's broken bone, if set properly, will heal. Likewise an otherwise healthy person with any of several kinds bacterial infections can be cured with antibiotics. The value of these treatments are easy to prove because they are nearly 100% effective. That is, if the appropriate antibiotic was administered to 1,000 otherwise healthy people with pneumococcal pneumonia for example, nearly all of them would have their pneumonia quickly eradicated. If another 1000 people with pneumococcal pneumonia received no antibiotic, many of them would not recover.

What's more, the effect of an antibiotic on various types of bacteria can be easily tested. The drug will either kill or not kill the bacteria.

With most cancer treatments though, the results are not nearly as clear. It is not at all unusual for a treatment to be partially effective for some patients, completely effective for others, and ineffective for others still. This makes the scientific proof much more complex than in a simple yes or no, all or nothing situation.

For any treatment claims to be considered valid, the same or similar results have to be achieved over and over again. If 10 people with colon cancer switched to the same macrobiotic diet, received no other treatment, and 9 of the 10 saw their cancer disappear, that would be a reasonable indication that the diet was at least partly responsible. If 1000 people with colon cancer switched to the same macrobiotic diet and 900 of them saw their cancer disappear, that would be an even better indication that the diet was responsible.

All reputable science relies on the scientific method. Whether the research is measuring the effectiveness of a new cancer treatment, the prospects of a political candidate, or consumer reaction to a new breakfast cereal the principles of scientific inquiry remain the same. While the methods differ, the underlying theory of research is quite straightforward as we'll see below.

Scientific Research

Understanding the basic concepts of scientific research is essential to making informed decisions about your care and treatment. Knowing that all sound medical treatment is based upon scientific research, and understanding what scientific research is about, will protect you from confusing supposition and unsubstantiated claims with valid care options.

Scientific research depends upon comparing various treatments to one another and to no treatment at all. The purpose of these comparisons is to determine whether each treatment works, how well it works, and whether each treatment is truly better than no treatment at all. In medical experimentation the subjects be they beakers filled with a specific substance, animals, or people, are divided into groups. Some of the groups receive the treatment being examined, some others do not. The no treatment group is called the control group. This group is used for comparison purposes: to compare the degree to which those in the treatment group(s) fare relative to those in the control group. Trying the treatment on groups of subjects is important in proving that it was the treatment that made the difference and that the cure or improvement was not coincidental.

The larger the treatment and control groups, the more likely it is that the results can be trusted. Also, the higher the percentages of patients in the treatment group who are helped, the more reliable the results. In the case of some rare diseases it is not possible to assemble a large treatment group. But if a treatment is highly effective, its value can still be scientifically demonstrated. The initial report in the New England Journal of Medicine on the drug that I received had only been administered to 12 patients with hairy cell leukemia. However, following treatment, 11 of those 12 were completely free of disease and the remaining 1 was markedly improved though not disease free. Further, the same drug was used on a much larger sample of patients with a different form of leukemia. While it was not as effective in combating that type of leukemia, these patients did not develop long terms side effects, indicating the drug was not likely to prove dangerous in terms of side effects.

Experimental treatment studies that show promise are always replicated. This simply means repeating the same treatment and control procedure again under the same conditions. More often than not, replication takes place not only at the facility where it was first tried, but in at least one other location as well. It is not unusual for the same treatment to be carried out at several locations concurrently.

Replication is done for the same reasons that studies are done with large groups of patients when possible; to make certain that the results are not coincidental, treatment is truly effective, and that the risks and side effects are outweighed by the potential benefits. Replication at another facility also lessens any potential for bias by researchers at any of the experimentation sites.

We are all familiar with seemingly promising medical findings reported in the media that are eventually shown to have much less promise once initial studies are replicated. During the 1970s a drug made from apricot pits called laetrile was touted as curative for several forms of cancer. Scientific replication eventually proved such claims to be, at best, overstated. In the 1980s, a substance called interferon that is naturally produced in the human body, was found to be effective in treating some forms of cancers when administered in large quantities. However, further study found interferon to be of more limited benefit than originally indicated.

The importance of basing medical decisions on research becomes clear when considering the alternative: basing decisions on anecdotal information. Anecdotes are isolated (and often very interesting and appealing) stories you will hear about what may have worked for your friend's brother or your aunt's neighbor's daughter who had the same condition that you have. It may be that eating seaweed with every meal worked for aunt's neighbor's daughter. It also may be that the seaweed had nothing to do with her recovery. That is, that the seaweed eating and her recovery was merely a coincidence. Finally, it may be that she had a different condition, and that her cure was based more on wishful thinking than upon medical verification. It's hard to know without scientific inquiry.

Understanding the basics of scientific inquiry can prove a powerful weapon in analyzing and understanding treatment possibilities. With a basic understanding of legitimate scientific research you will at least know which possibilities deserve further consideration and which are merely unproven hypothesis, bids for publicity, or cruel hoaxes. If you don't insist that a proposed treatment's scientific basis be demonstrated, the persuasive powers of the source of the information, and your own biases will have too much influence upon what you accept as valid.

How Clinical Trials Work

There are well over 1100 clinical trials taking place in the United States at any given time. Reputable clinical trials take place in other nation's throughout the world as well. In this and in virtually all other developed nations, a new drug must be extensively tested and evaluated in laboratories and then on animals, before it is used for humans.

Virtually all U.S. clinical trials are performed only with the approval of the U.S. Food and Drug Administration (FDA) and according to strict FDA guidelines. Also, most clinical trials must first be approved by an Institutional Review Board (IRB) at the institution where the trial is to take place. The IRB, which is composed of physicians, scientists, and others reviews the study to assure that it is well designed and that it includes appropriate safeguards for the patients, and that the potential benefits outweigh the potential risks. Clinical trials are carefully reviewed for medical ethics, patient safety, and scientific merit by the organization that is sponsoring the research. As with the practice of medicine in general, a key ethical tenant must be observed: nothing shall be done to a patient that will knowingly do any harm that is not outweighed by a greater benefit.

A clinical trial must have a clear and potentially helpful purpose with clear evaluation criteria and clear steps in its administration. In many instances effectiveness in destroying or abating cancer relative to standard therapies is being tested. In some cases effectiveness of two or more drugs has been proven to be similar but relative toxicities (peripheral damage caused by treatment) need to be evaluated.

While the heavy scrutiny that a clinical trial receives does not guarantee that every trial is absolutely safe, it is at least very significant protection against carelessness and undue risk under the circumstances. In all cases you will receive information about the potential benefits and hazards and you will not be admitted to a clinical trial until and unless you consent in writing to be part of that trial. Even with your written consent, you can leave the clinical trial at any time and for any reason or for no reason at all.

Clinical Trial Phases

Trials in cancer research in this country are designed in three key phases with each phase building upon what was learned in the previous phase. Not all trials make it through all three phases if the value is called into question by early data. Also, some clinical trials are allowed to forego phase 3 if earlier results are particularly promising. The phases are outlined as follows:

Phase I
Logically enough, the first clinical trial phase is called phase I. In this phase a new drug is first administered to humans. Because the drug

is new to humans, risks are highest here. Part of the researchers job is to determine the best way to administer the drug, appropriate dosage, and of course to carefully monitor side effects. Only people with advanced disease who could not be helped by other known treatment are typically allowed to participate in this potentially perilous phase.

Phase II
A drug that shows clear signs of effectiveness without undue risk of damage enters the next phase of human trial. In this phase, access is opened up to more patients. Unlike with phase one of a trial, it is no longer limited to those with advance disease who can not be helped by more established treatments. However, other restrictions on eligibility may, and often do apply. Patients with forms of cancer related to the specific cancer the trial was designed for in phase1, may be admitted into phase II trials.

Phase III
The key to this phase is comparison of the new treatment with other treatments. The group getting the new treatment is called the treatment group and the group getting the standard treatment is called the control group. Where there is no existing treatment, the treatment group gets the treatment and the control group gets no treatment at all. In these situations, the control group instead gets a placebo which is a non-drug substance that looks exactly the same as the drug being administered to the treatment group. Patients are randomly assigned to the treatment or control group through a process called randomization. While this is good science it unfortunately means some patients get a treatment that may not be as good as other patients are getting. For this reason, the FDA sometimes permits this phase to be skipped if there is clear evidence that the investigational treatment is better than the existing alternatives (or lack thereof).

Before a drug is approved by the FDA as a standard treatment, that agency reviews all the clinical trial data. This is a lengthy process taking at least a year and sometimes much more. In fact, it can easily take 5 to 10 years from the point where an investigational drug is first administered to a patient to the time it is fully approved by the FDA.

NCI Group C Treatment Protocols

Group C treatments are drugs provided to physicians by the NCI for treatment of individual patients. Drugs in this category, although still in clinical trial, have been FDA approved for treatment of specific cancers. They have passed through extensive clinical trials (at least through phase II.) and show considerable promise. If all goes according to expectation with a drug in this group, it will soon be approved for commercialization.

Patient Follow Up in Clinical Trials

Just about all cancer survivors are closely followed with frequent tests and evaluation. Patients who participate in clinical trials are followed even more closely. The researchers and the FDA demand precise data as part of the trial. Of course, the need for patient data does not end with the treatment. It is crucial to know how a patient is doing months and years after treatment has ended. Of course patients retain the right to refuse these follow up test but most accept them as a contribution to scientific knowledge.

Costs of Clinical Trials

Costs to the patient of clinical trials range from no cost at all to sums that are beyond the means of all but the wealthiest patients. Institutional policies differ as to compensation arrangements to the institutions conducting the studies. Some are wholly or partly supported by grants, other are not. Often the drug itself is free, but charges for its administration and peripheral hospital services must be born by the patient.

To complicate matters further, many health insurance policies do not cover clinical trials. Some won't cover the clinical trial itself but will cover the peripheral medical services. Before calling your health insurance carrier it might be a good idea to talk with your lawyer about how or whether to handle such an inquiry.

If you want to enter a particular clinical trial but can not afford it, check with the hospital or clinic social service office, the NCI

Cancer Information Service (1-800-4-CANCER), or the local American Cancer Society chapter. One of these offices may be able to direct you to help.

If you still can't pay for needed services talk to your lawyer about an appropriate strategy. There may be steps you can take that would be unpleasant, such as declaring personal bankruptcy, but better than depriving yourself of life saving treatment.

Should You Participate In a Clinical Trial?

On the whole, far more people have been helped than hurt by clinical trials conducted in this country. Trials are carefully scrutinized by the FDA and by institutional review boards. Precautionary steps are taken to offer reasonable assurance that the potential risks to participants are outweighed by the potential benefits. Clinical trials definitely offer the latest developments in cancer treatment, and quite possibly offer the best treatments as well.

Nevertheless, clinical trials are not for every one. While steps are taken to protect participating patients, clinical trials have their risks. A treatment can prove to be effective in the short run but not in the long run. Later side effects too, are a possibility. Finally, entry into a clinical trial often means temporarily or permanently forgoing standard treatment. The safety and effectiveness of your standard treatment options, of course, have to be weighed against the indicated safety and effectiveness of the clinical trial option(s).

The FDA is often criticized for being too slow in approving new drugs. However, the purpose of insisting on thorough clinical trial is to assess the risk versus the benefit of new treatments. Without such safeguards, there is the real possibility that a new drug will become readily available only to later be shown to be more dangerous than its benefits justify.

It is important that you find out about all your options and evaluate for yourself whether a clinical trial, a standard treatment, or no treatment is in your own best interest. There is no absolute right choice for every patient. The patient with the best information will make the best personal decision.

Finding Out About Clinical Trials

Ask Your Doctor

Your initial doctor or the doctor who you see for a second opinion may know about clinical trials in progress. However, don't assume that the doctor will automatically share whatever knowledge he has about clinical trials if you don't ask. Some doctors are biased against sending their patients to trials and some assume that patients don't want to be in trials. Be sure you ask each doctor you consult if he has heard of any clinical trials that might be appropriate for you.

National Cancer Institute

The NCI's Cancer Information Service can look into clinical trials that are being conducted for your specific disease. Call their 1-800-4-CANCER phone helpline and they will check into it for you. If the NCI staff person finds clinical trials that are going on, a printout(s) with a description of the trial, the institution where it is taking place, the name of the lead researcher, criteria for entering the trial, and other information will be sent to you.

Physician's Data Query (PDQ)

The NCI's public information service relies largely on the PDQ data base for information on clinical trials. This database, which is constantly updated, has information about over 1100 clinical trial in progress. If you prefer, you can access the database directly through your own computer. This database, and ways to access it, are explained in chapter eight.

Cancer Associations

Foundations and associations dedicated to your specific type of illness often collect and disseminate information on clinical trials. They may in fact have some information about potential upcoming trials before they are underway and therefore before they have been entered into PDQ. Call the appropriate association(s) and ask if they know about current or upcoming clinical trials. Appendix IV lists several cancer associations.

Foreign Clinical Trials

While some foreign clinical trials may be included on PDQ, many others are not. One systematic way to find out about treatments throughout the world is through a European maintained medical database service known as Embase. This database is not accessed by the NCI information personnel. It is accessible in this country but not as easily as the U.S. based databases. It is discussed in the next section.

Schine On-line Services

As an outgrowth of this book, I have set up a company that searches the medical databases in the U.S. and throughout the world on behalf of cancer patients. Our service provides information on clinical trials and on recent findings about any form of cancer. Our services are described in the last chapter.

"Unapproved Drugs"

According to the FDA, unapproved drugs are drugs which have not been proven in terms of safety or efficacy. There are some drugs that are unapproved because they have failed to achieve FDA standards for safety and efficacy. Such drugs are generally prohibited for use in the U.S.. There are other drugs, however, which have good scientific indication of efficacy and safety which have not yet made it through the lengthy FDA approval process. Though unapproved by the FDA, such drugs are not necessarily unsafe, ineffective, unavailable to you, or illegal to use.

Before getting involved with unapproved drugs, it is important to understand that you are taking some risk. The FDA is very careful when it comes to approving drugs for general use; probably more careful than its counterpart agencies anywhere in the world. While the FDA's screen might screen out some safe drugs, it also assuredly screens out some drugs that carry more risk than a drug should. In accepting unapproved treatment, you are bypassing a screen. Don't do this without first doing your homework and looking into the treatment's track record for effectiveness and possible dangers.

Unapproved drug treatments that can be used in this country fall into two broad categories, as explained below.

Drugs Approved For Another Purpose

Typically, when a drug has completed clinical trial and is federally approved, it is approved for one or for a very few specific illnesses. Pharmaceutical companies manufacturing that drug can market it only for its approved purpose(s). However, once that drug is available to them, physicians are not prohibited from using it for other illnesses on a patient by patient basis.

It is not at all unusual that a drug approved for one type of cancer will later be shown effective for a related form of cancer. It is less common but not unheard of that a drug will be proven effective for an unrelated form of cancer as well.

Journal articles and other cancer literature are filled with articles about approved drugs being tested for other cancers with varying degrees of success. Finding such articles may point you in the direction of an unapproved but effective treatment. The next chapter (Chapter eight) details ways in which you can search the latest research available in the hope that you will find a drug that has helped people with your specific illness.

The fact that a drug is approved for human use indicates that it meets FDA guidelines for safety, at least for the approved purpose. This implies, but by no means does it guarantee, the drug's safety for unapproved uses.

Despite the FDA tolerance, physicians and hospital administrators are sometimes reluctant to use approved drugs in unapproved ways. The risk of liability and malpractice suits is a genuine concern to them. If a physician agrees to treat you with a substance not approved for your illness, expect to be asked to sign forms releasing the doctor and the hospital from liability.

Also, the use of approved substances in unapproved ways may not always be so easy. The FDA has, on occasion considered clamping down on this practice. As of now though, it is not unusual for patients to be treated, and helped, with drugs that are not specifically approved for their illness.

Drugs Approved For Use In Foreign Countries, But Not Approved Here

Drugs that are approved for use in a foreign nation that are not specifically prohibited in the U.S., may generally be used for treatment here. However, they may not be easily obtained here.

An individual may bring up to a three month supply of such a medication into the U.S. for personal use if that individual has a prescription for the medication from a U.S. physician. So, you are permitted to get a doctor's prescription, go to another country, buy the appropriate medication, and bring it back here for your own use. If treatment is actually started in a foreign country, a prescription from a physician in that country is also acceptable for importing medication for personal use

There are two sources to check for foreign approved drugs that might be helpful to you. The first is a book called *Drugs Available Abroad- A Guide to Therapeutic Drugs Available and Approved Outside the United States.* The other is the Embase computerized database. The *Drugs Available Abroad* book is listed in appendix V. Embase is discussed in the next chapter (chapter eight).

Finally, before embarking on any foreign pharmaceutical ventures, check with your attorney. You have to make sure that you do it right and that no state or federal laws or laws of foreign countries will be an obstacle to your mission. ❖

❖

Finding The Latest Information Available About Your Illness

C hapter two detailed some of the ways that you can find basic information about your specific kind of cancer. This chapter explains some of the more sophisticated searching techniques and sources for locating the most current information including clinical trials, evaluations of those trials, other current findings, and information regarding specific physicians and their research.

Few practicing physicians have the time to keep up to date on more than a few of the latest developments in specific cancer treatments. You as the patient, however, have the option of gathering the information that can give you a better chance at a longer life. Your best chance of learning about new developments is by taking responsibility for doing the researching on your own.

Much of the information that comes from the steps explained in this chapter is technical in nature and will need to be interpreted by a physician. Your job is to find the information and bring it to the attention of someone who can interpret it and determine whether it is appropriate in your particular situation. Keep in mind however that physicians differ in the way they view new treatments. If you uncover something that you believe is appropriate, but your doctor thinks that it is not, don't hesitate to get another opinion (See chapter six on the need for a second opinion). Finally, note that most articles and studies that you locate will have the names of the author(s) and the researching physicians involved in the study. Don't hesitate to call those doctors and ask them whether the treatment might be right for you.

Organization of this Chapter

Until recently, research of medical literature was primarily carried out through printed books and periodicals in libraries. Since the mid

1970s, computers have made gradual inroads into this type of medical research. Today, much research is achieved through computerized databases which have a lot of advantages over the more traditional methods. This chapter first explains the various sources where you can access printed information. Next it explains the mechanics and advantages of accessing information via personal computer. Finally, specific resources are described along with availability and methods of access whether they be by print, by computer, or by both.

Libraries

Much medical information is available through libraries although the best libraries for researching your illness, are probably not the ones with which you are most familiar.

General Libraries

Major metropolitan libraries will have some of the resources discussed in this chapter. Smaller community libraries will have very few of them. If you live near a major library, by all means pay that library a visit first. Otherwise, go right to one of the next kinds of libraries described below.

Hospital Libraries

Many major hospitals have their own medical libraries, some of which are excellent facilities with helpful personnel. Access policies range from "staff use only" to "open to the public." In some cases, patients (including transient outpatients) are allowed access to that hospital's library although the general public may not be. Call the larger hospitals in your area and ask for the library. Ask the librarian about access policies. If it is closed to you, ask which local medical libraries are open to the public. If none are, ask about exceptions to the restricted access policies.

Some private libraries share their resources with other libraries in the community. In practice, this means that the public library may be able to issue you a pass to a hospital library if you are looking for an item not available in that public library. Ask the public or hospital librarian.

Medical School Libraries

Medical schools have their own medical libraries. Again, access policies differ. State run medical school libraries are usually open to the public whereas private medical school libraries may not be. Call and ask.

State Department of Health Libraries

Most states have at least one department of health library and most of those are open to the public (at least to state residents).

National Cancer Institute:
Cancer Information Service Libraries

There are twenty-one regional NCI libraries in the U.S.. The Cancer Information Service (described in chapter two) does most of its work via telephone call-in through their 1-800-4-CANCER line. Although the NCI doesn't publicize the fact, its regional libraries are open to the public. Holdings are limited primarily to NCI material, some material from cancer associations and societies, and the PDQ and Cancerlit databases. Call 1-800-4-CANCER and ask where the NCI regional library nearest to you is located.

Medical Consumer Libraries

There are at least two medical consumer libraries in the U.S.. One, the Center for Medical Consumers, is located in New York City. The other, Planetree Health Resource Center is in San Fransisco. Planetree also has a specialty bookstore within their facility (Planetree Books). Both libraries offer books, periodicals, and articles that may be helpful. Since these libraries are geared toward non-physicians, they tend to be less intimidating and more user friendly. Their staffs are also more helpful and more in-tune with the patient's level of knowledge, and the patient's information needs.

Their addresses are:

Center for Medical Consumers
237 Thompson Street
New York, NY 10012
(212) 674-7105

Planetree Health Resource Center
2040 Webster Street
San Fransisco, CA 94115
(415) 923-3680

Computers and Research

In medicine as in most fields, computer databases are rapidly becoming the standard method of finding information. Just a few years ago researching the latest findings took a major medical library and hours of laboriously researching. Today, if you have a telephone, computer, modem, and the right inexpensive software, you have easy access to a wealth of current information about your condition, your treatment options, and more.*

Basics of Searching Electronic Databases

In essence, medical information in the form of articles, summaries of articles, details on clinical trials, and other information is stored in computer memory by the organizations maintaining the database(s). Updates are typically added at regular and frequent intervals, weekly in many instances. The computers storing the information, called host computers, are set up to communicate with other computers and provide access to the data they hold.

The host computers can be accessed by virtually any desktop computer over standard telephone lines. You simply call a special local access number or an 800 number to tap the host computer's memory, wherever that host may be. Through your computer, you can communicate with the host computer, request information from it, and save (capture) that information into your computer's memory.

Of course, even though the host computer has a huge memory, it has no brain. Therefore, you must be precise in telling it what information to retrieve. The machine can not help you limit your search or make intelligent suggestions as to what you should be looking for. If you ask for information on skin cancer, it will dutifully send your computer hundreds of pages of information on skin cancer leaving you to sift through it all and pay a bill that is based on time

---

* *If you don't want to get involved with searching via computers yourself, but you want it done for you, see section 9.*

connected and information retrieved. Therefore, it is important that your search be limited as precisely as possible so as to retrieve information that is most relevant to your needs. Using keywords and other limiting techniques which are explained later in this chapter, are therefore necessary.

Equipment You'll Need

Besides a computer, you will need three basic items to access a computerized database: a modem, software to run the modem, and a password issued by the organization that offers the database or provides access to it.

Modem — A modem is a device that permits a computer to communicate with other computers over phone lines. It connects to your computer and to a telephone jack. Some computers have modems built in, others require an external modem. Hooking an external modem to a computer is usually quite easy. Hooking the modem to a telephone line is as simple as plugging it into a phone jack exactly as you would plug in a telephone. A basic (and perfectly usable) modem will cost between $90 and $200.

Software — Software is what tells a computer what to do and how to do it. You will need communication software that tells your computer and modem how to communicate with distant computers and how to capture the information that you want to extract from that computer.

There are several communication software packages on the market that can be used to enable your computer to communicate with just about any other computer. However, if you are new to computer communication and your interest in it is limited to researching your illness, you are better off buying a communication package called *Grateful Med*. This package, sold by the National Library of Medicine for $29.95, makes using the all-important NLM databases quite easy. The only real problems with this software is that the ease of use means you sacrifice some searching flexibility, and you can only use it to access the NLM databases. It can not be used to access any other databases the way commercial software can. Grateful Med is explained further later in this chapter.

Password — This is simply a word or number that identifies you to the host computer primarily for billing purposes. It can be obtained from the database provider sometimes for free and sometimes for an upfront fee. In either case, you are charged for use every time your password is used to gather information on-line. Most database providers offer a small amount of free on-line time with a new password so you can practice using the database service without running up a bill.

Advantages of Searching By Computer

The advantages of searching by computer are formidable:

Access from Anywhere — If you have a computer you can do your research from anywhere that you can connect up to a standard telephone line. Gone are the days when a researcher needed access to major big city libraries. From your office desktop or your kitchen table, you can gain the same access to the same medical databases that researchers at the nation's top hospital and research facilities have.

Search by Keywords — Computer searches can be done by keywords and phrases which can be linked so only articles containing your chosen key words are included in your search. Suppose, for example, that you suffer from a large cell lymphoma and want information on bone marrow transplants for that illness. Suppose further that you have all the information you need that was reported before January of 1992. You can instruct the computer to retrieve only articles that contain the words "large cell lymphoma," "marrow," and "transplant" that were published after December of 1991. In seconds, the computer can search thousands of articles and reports and give you only those that contain all the selected words that were published after December 1991.

Once you get the hang of it, searching for specific information this way is far more efficient than the old way of going to the library, searching indexes and then searching for articles.

Continuous Updating — Computer databases are continually updated. There is no need to wait for the new edition of a medical journal or a medical index to be released. This can cut several weeks or months off the time it takes for you to find information about an important development.

Around the Clock Access — Electronic databases are available virtually 24 hours a day. While some are down for maintenance or updating periodically, such gaps in service are typically only a few hours and only once weekly or less.

No Missing or In-Use Material — Who hasn't tried to get a book or article from the library only to learn it was lost, stolen, or in use by another patron? This doesn't happen with electronic databases. The information doesn't really leave the computer where it is stored. Rather, it is copied by the computer that is requesting it from the host computer so it is never missing and can be used by several users at the same time.

Disadvantages of Searching By Computer

There are a few disadvantages to searching for information via computer:

Equipment — A pen, notebook, and a handful of change for a coin operated copying machine, is all the equipment you need to competently do library research. To search electronic databases you need the equipment outlined above such as a computer, modem, and software. If you already have most of this equipment, this disadvantage doesn't apply. If you have access to none of it, you're looking at an obstacle of at least $1,500.

You Need To Know How To Search By Computer — If you are reasonably computer literate, this will not be a major problem. Searching by computer, especially with Grateful Med, is not difficult for a person with a modest amount of computer experience. However, if you're not comfortable with computer use, you do face a learning curve.

Cost — Using electronic databases is not cheap. Costs have come down and may continue to fall, but searching this way can be expensive. This is especially true if you are not an experienced searcher. It takes a while to get the hang of it and while you are learning and searching, the meter is running.

Mechanics of Gathering Information On-line

Modems and communication software come with instructions on setting up the hardware and software. While there are some initial set-up technicalities, getting your hardware and software ready shouldn't take more than an hour, even if you are new to computer telecommunications.

In the actual communication with a host computer, there are three basic methods for telling that computer what information you are looking to retrieve from it. Some databases can be accessed by only one of the three methods while others are accessible by two or three of them. The methods of access for each database discussed in this chapter are noted with each discussion. The three basic methods are:

Command Language

People experienced in computer telecommunication use a system of commands that precisely tell a host computer what to do. The commands are a type of language devised strictly for the purpose of retrieving information from computer databases. Of the three methods outlined here, command languages offer the most power and flexibility. If you are familiar with the relevant languages, this is the best way to get all the information you're looking for without also getting a good deal of unwanted information along with it.

However, command languages are not for the novice user. Firstly, learning a command language well enough to use it competently takes time, at least days and quite possibly weeks. If you don't know the language used by the database(s) you're trying to use, you can't fake it. The following interaction for example between the NLM computer system and a user would mean nothing to some one not trained in NLM command language:

SS 1 /C?
USER:
explode eye
Prog:
MM (EYE) (2)
      1. A1.456.505.420
      2. A9.371
Number, NONE, OR EXPAND

Further, command languages are not tolerant of seemingly minor discrepancies. For example the use of a colon instead of a semicolon or a period instead of a comma can mean the difference between a host computer dutifully executing your search and sending back a message telling you it has no idea what you want it to do.

Finally, the languages differ from one database to the next. Commands for Embase for example, while related to those for Cancerlit, are not the same. To use command language for these two databases, the user would have to have familiarity with both languages.

If you are new to searching computer databases on-line, and your only interest in on-line searching is to research your illness, I recommend you don't get involved with command searching. Fortunately, there are alternatives for the non-professional searchers.

Menus

Years ago, the people who operated computer databases realized that, as long as their databases could only be accessed through command language, their growth would be very limited. To partly solve this problem, they developed menu driven access software.

Menus, as the name implies, give the user choices as to what to do. The host computer offers several choices with a number preceding each choice. The user then chooses the number for his choice which may lead to several additional menus that serve to further limit the search. Bank automatic teller machines are a common form of communicating with a computer through menus. When you use a bank ATM, you are given a series of menus from which you can instruct the computer as to the transaction you wish to carry out. It may look like this:

What would you like to do?

1. Make a deposit
2. Withdraw funds
3. Make a loan payment
4. Get account information

If you choose "2. Withdraw funds", you will be given a new menu asking for example:

Withdraw funds from:

1. Savings account
2. Checking account

After making your choice you will then be asked how much you want to withdraw, etc.

Most on-line databases offer more options than bank ATM's so their menus have more choices. Nevertheless the principles are quite similar. Physician's Data Query (PDQ), discussed later in this chapter, is a menu driven database. Here is a sample interaction between the PDQ database and a user:

SO THAT PDQ CAN SEND YOU INFORMATION IN THE PROPER WAY, PLEASE INDICATE HOW YOU WOULD LIKE YOUR OUTPUT DISPLAYED:

1 CONTINUOUSLY. PDQ SENDS INFORMATION WITHOUT PAUSES

2 ONE PAGE OR UNIT OF INFORMATION AT A TIME.

3 HELP. EXPLAINS MORE ABOUT 1 AND 2 ABOVE.
ENTER 1, 2 OR 3 —> 1

AFTER YOU SEE THE PROMPT (>)
TYPE "START" AND PRESS CR (RETURN KEY) TO BEGIN, OR
TYPE "END" AND PRESS CR IF YOU DO NOT WISH TO CONTINUE
::
>start

NXM.USER.GED24.DATA   ON PRIV85 AS SGED24 SEQ OLD

THE NATIONAL LIBRARY OF MEDICINE WELCOMES YOU TO
THE NATIONAL CANCER INSTITUTE'S PDQ SYSTEM

Date: 11/21/92   Time: 8:56 PM EST
 Cancer screening guidelines have been added to PDQ; select Cancer
Information from the main PDQ menu, then Cancer Screening
Guidelines from the submenu.

For information about the Breast Cancer Prevention Trial (BCPT),
drugs available from the NCI through the Group C mechanism, or
NCI high priority clinical trials, see the PDQ News.

*Press CR to continue.
>

            PDQ MENU

The following information is available in PDQ.

1 Information about PDQ   5 Physicians
2 PDQ Editorial Board   6 Organizations
3 News   7 Protocols
4 Cancer Information   8 CANCERLIT Searches
            9 Exit PDQ

At any PDQ prompt (>), you may type HELP to obtain assistance with your
PDQ search.

*Enter desired number and press CR ("Return" or "Enter" key).

>4

PDQ: look up cancer information

1 Treatment by body system/site
2 Treatment by histologic tissue/type
3 Treatment of childhood cancer

4 Supportive care
5 Rare tumor
6 Cancer screening guidelines
7 Design of clinical trials

*Enter desired number OR type in a diagnosis and press CR.

>hairy cell leukemia

Searching...
HAIRY CELL LEUKEMIA retrieved 1 diagnosis

CANCER INFORMATION MENU

HAIRY CELL LEUKEMIA

Information for Patients   State-of-the-Art Information
_____   _____

                         4 Prognosis
1 Description   5 Cellular Classification
2 Stage Explanations   6 Stage Information
3 General Treatment Options   7 Treatment by Cell Type/Stage

              8 Display all information
              9 Continuation options for citation abstracts,
                CANCERLIT searches and protocols

*Enter desired number and press CR.

>8
          PRINT OPTIONS FOR CANCER INFORMATION

HAIRY CELL LEUKEMIA
1 Display all Information for Patients (1-3)

2 Display all State-of-the-Art Information (4-7)
3 Display all Information (1-7)
4 Return to the Cancer Information Menu

*Enter desired number and press CR.
>3

Menu driven software opens the world of on-line databases to novice users. The ease of use does come with a price though. Menus offer less flexibility and less precision for instructing the host computer to send exactly and exclusively the information for which you are looking. Recently for example, I needed information from the Embase database (discussed later in this chapter). Embase can be accessed either through menus or command language. The information I wanted from it involved studies on treatments for large cell lymphoma that were neither carried out in the United States nor reported in a U.S. medical journal. The menus didn't come close to allowing me this kind of searching precision. Through the command language, getting the information I was after took only a few minutes.

If I did not know how to use Embase via commands, I could have used the menus and received a good deal of what I was looking for along with a good deal of superfluous information. That is, I could easily limit my search to large cell lymphoma treatment through the menus, but not limit to non U.S. origination and non U.S. journals. I would have had to pay for the superfluous information and would have needed to sift through dozens of pages of information to choose only the information I needed, a task the computer did for me quicker, cheaper, and better.

Dedicated Access Software

Most of the software packages used for computer telecommunications can be used for virtually any database. However, some packages are designed to access a single database or group of databases. The limitation to a single system of databases is made up for in ease of use.

The premier dedicated software package for searching medical databases is called Grateful Med. It can be used to easily search many of the important National library of Medicine on-line databases such as Medline, Cancerlit, and SDIline, all of which are described below.

Grateful Med makes access to much of the NLM's Medlars system, the world's most important system of medical databases, very easy. This software is even more impressive when you consider that the command language for accessing the NLM computers is, by today's standards, complex, unforgiving, and antiquated.

Once the initial set-up is completed, a task which will take less than an hour, Grateful Med will help you compose an effective search, call the NLM computer, perform the search, and hang up when the search is complete.

As good as Grateful Med is, it does have its limitations. First, it does not have the flexibility of command language. Also, if you don't understand the NLM's esoteric vocabulary called MeSH (which stands for Medical Subject Headings) your use of the NLM databases is limited and the risk of omissions and inappropriate retrievals is considerable. Nevertheless, if you are inexperienced with searching databases via computer, you don't want to spend days or weeks learning to use commands, but you do want to use the on-line medical databases, this is by far your best option.

To order Grateful Med, see the section below on the National Library of Medicine.

Searching Databases via CD ROM

Some of the databases available on-line are also available on CD-ROM. While CD-ROM disks look like CDs for your home stereo, they are actually very high capacity storage devices for computer readable information. It doesn't make sense for an individual patient to purchase CD-ROM for seeking medical information. The purchase price is prohibitive, when compared to the amount of on-line charges that you are likely to run-up even for exhaustive searches.

However, purchasing database access via CD-ROM makes a great deal of sense for libraries and other facilities that use databases heavily. Unlike online service, the subscriber pays a flat fee for initial purchase and periodic updating, not for each use. The purchase and updating costs can be more than offset by savings in on-line charges. Many libraries do use CD-ROM because of the economic advantage. Those that do are understandably more willing to let you search a CD-ROM than to let you run up their on-line bill.

Typically, a subscriber receives periodic CD-ROM updates with the latest information. While the updating is usually quite good, CD-ROM's by nature are not as current as their on-line counterparts.

If a database is currently available on CD ROM, it is so noted in the discussion of that database below. More and more databases are being released in this format. By the time you read this chapter, there may well be databases available on CD ROM that are not currently available through this medium.

Accessing The Databases

There are a number of separate databases available that contain highly current cancer information. Although the databases are separate, nearly all of them can be accessed through one of three services that are outlined below. In fact, since the three overlap in their offerings, if you arrange access to either Dialog, Medlars or CompuServe, you then have access to most of the important databases.

National Library of Medicine (MEDLARS)

Most of the medical databases in this chapter— in fact most of the medical databases available period— are available on-line through the National Library of Medicine's Medlars service. Medlars includes more than 15 different medical databases.

Through the Grateful Med software package (described above), access to Medlars databases is quite easy, even for the less sophisticated computer user. To access Medlars directly, you will need to open an account and obtain a password. There is no fee for opening the account nor is there a monthly fee. You are charged based only upon use.

Unless you are versed in accessing databases through command language, you will also need the Grateful Med package which is available for both IBM compatible and Macintosh computers for $29.95 plus $3.00 for shipping.

MEDLARS offers very competent telephone support for on-line users. There is no limit to the amount of free help you receive; in fact, they don't even ask for your name, password, or account number when you phone their 800 number with questions.

To order a password and open an account with Medlars write or call:

Medlars Management Section
National Library of Medicine
Bethesda, MD 20894
1-800-638-8480

To purchase Grateful Med write or call:
U.S. Department of Commerce
National Technical Information Service
Springfield, VA 22161
(703)-487-4650

Getting both a password and the Grateful Med program will take about a week.

CompuServe

CompuServe is a sort of information mall. Through CompuServe, you can access all kinds of information from any computer with a modem. CompuServe includes two of the key government sponsored databases, Medline and Physician's Data Query (PDQ). Both of these are also available through Medlars. CompuServe is, as of this writing, the exclusive on-line access system for the National Organization for Rare Disorders (NORD) database.

Unlike Medlars, you can sign up for CompuServe immediately by calling 1-800-848-8199 and billing to your credit card. The current price is $39.95 for initial sign-up, which includes a $25 usage credit. CompuServe also charges a monthly fee of $7.95. Medline and PDQ carry additional charges for their use, NORD does not. Both Medline and PDQ are markedly cheaper and easier to use through Medlars and Grateful Med. However, if you are already a CompuServe user, if you absolutely can't wait to sign up for Medlars, or if you want on-line access to NORD, CompuServe may be the way to go.

Dialog

Dialog is another on-line vendor of many databases from many different fields. Dialog is designed more for organizational use than individual use. It is generally harder and more expensive to use than CompuServe and Medlars. However, if you are already a Dialog user or know someone who is, you should know that it includes several medical databases including some of the ones covered below (as noted).

One important Dialog database offering that is not available through Medlars or CompuServe is Embase, a European based outfit. Embase is very strong in drug related treatment research and in non U.S. clinical trials and studies. Embase is described more fully below.

Dialog also markets a sort of junior version of its services known as Knowledge Index. KI includes only some of the full Dialog collection of databases, but it does include Cancerlit, Medline , and Embase. Unlike the standard service, you can sign up for Knowledge Index by phone with a credit card. This service is restricted to use between six p.m. and five a.m. your local time. The initial fee is $40.00 which includes two free hours of use. For information on Dialog and to sign up for its Knowledge Index service, call 1-800-334-2564 or 415-858-3785.

The remainder of this chapter explains specific print and computer information resources along with information on finding and accessing each resource.

Physician's Data Query (PDQ)

This menu driven database, maintained by the National Cancer Institute, was conceived as a vehicle to bring the latest in cancer information and treatment options to physicians who treat cancer. Many comprehensive and clinical care hospitals and clinics do indeed use the database for the purpose it was conceived. Unfortunately, it is unusual to find it being used in the offices of practicing physicians where it appropriately belongs.

PDQ is also used extensively by the NCI's Cancer Information Service (1-800-4-CANCER) to provide patients with general information about cancer and about standard treatments and clinical trials. The database is menu-driven. That is, it offers the user a series of menus with choices by numbers.

Some of the information you can find on PDQ includes:

❖ Detailed summaries of all major cancer types including prognosis, staging, cellular classifications, and state of the art treatment options.

❖ Information on over 1,000 active clinical trials with details on objectives of the trial and patient eligibility requirements. Information on clinical trials also includes the names and addresses for the principal researchers involved in each trial.

❖ Information on approximately 13,000 physicians who devote part or all of their practice to cancer. Data on each clinical trial in which each physician is involved is included.

PDQ divides some of its information into menu categories labeled "patient information" and "state of the art information." Chances are if you are reading this guide and have gotten this far, you'll be primarily interested in the state of the art information. The patient information is quite basic.

Accessing PDQ

This database is widely available through a variety of channels.

NCI-Cancer Information Service

When you call the NCI's **1-800-4-CANCER** service, much of the information that you'll receive is from PDQ. The information specialists refer to it for general information about your illness, as well as for information on clinical trials for which you may be a candidate. Accessing PDQ this way is free. Further, the NCI information specialists are versed in using PDQ so they may get more complete information more quickly than a novice user would.

On the downside, accessing PDQ through the NCI means that you are limited to receiving only what the person you speak to deems appropriate. If you search on your own, you can gather whatever information you want. You may be able to partially get around this problem by visiting one of the NCI Cancer Information Service offices personally and asking one of the staff people to search PDQ while you are there. You may also be able to watch and ask that he chooses specific choices that appear on the screen menu.

Another problem with PDQ through NCI is that most of its offices access the database not on-line but via in-office CD-ROM. This means that the very latest information may not be included. The information is only as current as their last CD-ROM update.

Medical Libraries

Many of the larger hospitals, medical school, and state health department libraries have PDQ access both on-line and on CD-ROM. While policies differ, few will allow you to search PDQ on-line at their expense. However, some librarians may search it for you. Others may let you search on CD-ROM and assist you with searching techniques.

CompuServe

You can access PDQ through CompuServe (give the command "GO PDQ" at any prompt). Accessing this way is expensive but if time is more scarce than money, it may be your best option, at least initially. As with other databases through CompuServe, you will be notified regarding current access fees before you are connected to PDQ. You will be given the option of canceling your request before surcharges start accruing.

MEDLARS (The National Library of Medicine)

This is the access method that I recommend. You can sign-on to PDQ quite easily and comparatively inexpensively through MEDLARS. The only problem is the delay of about a week in obtaining a password and the Grateful Med software package that is essential for all but experienced users.

Fax Machine

Through a new NCI service called Cancerfax, any one with access to a fax machine can get the PDQ patient information statement or physician statement. The PDQ clinical trial information is not available through Cancerfax.

To use this service, call 1-301-402-5874 from a fax telephone. You will be asked to make a few choices, such as whether you want information in English or Spanish, by pressing different numbers on your telephone. The first item you'll need is the list of codes (which changes monthly) for every type of cancer in the PDQ system and for other information. Press the appropriate number when prompted and the codes will be faxed to you immediately. You can then call back, enter the appropriate code and out comes your information.

According to NCI, Cancerfax is meant for physician use. They don't encourage patient use, but they don't prohibit it. The NCI press officer that I talked to explained, "If patients use the system, doctors may call and get a busy signal. Beside, patients don't want to know things like survival rates, it may upset them."

If you're not afraid of putting a physician at risk of getting a busy signal and you're not afraid to learn survival rates for the type of cancer you have, this is an easy and cheap way to get good initial information. The only charge is the phone call to Bethesda, Maryland.

InfoTrac

Unless your high school years were very recent, you probably were taught to find periodical articles by using a bound and printed index such as Reader's Guide to Periodical Literature. Such paper indexes are rapidly being replaced by higher technology CD-ROM based indexes. The index device uses a machine, essentially a personal computer with a CD-ROM reader. The CD-ROM disk itself is updated periodically.

InfoTrac, the most common of these CD-ROM indexes, is very easy to use, even to those who know nothing about computers. It is a sort of mega-index to periodicals covering a myriad of subjects including health and medicine. What's more, the index contains abstracts of some indexed articles and it will print the reference and abstract at the press of a button. Some of the articles can even be found in full text through a microfilm device that is an adjunct to the InfoTrac machine.

Looking up your illness on this index is certainly worthwhile. The general InfoTrac indexes do not include every professional medical journal but they do include the better known ones such as *The New England Journal of Medicine*. Unlike most of the indexes and databases explained in this chapter, this one is geared toward general reading so the abstracts are easily understandable to the lay person.

InfoTrac Health Reference Center

There is a specialized InfoTrac index for the health field. The Health Reference Center index includes articles from both professional and popular health periodicals. For more involved research into your illness, this index is more likely to be helpful.

Accessing InfoTrac
The general index is available at an increasing number of general and college libraries. It is designed to be used by the public so, if the library has it, getting access to it is not a problem.

Accessing InfoTrac Health Reference Center
This index is on a separate disk that is more likely to be found in a medical library than a general library. Currently, it is more the exception than the rule for medical libraries to have it, but more and more are obtaining it. It is worth searching for. Call any of your local medical libraries and ask if they have it. If they do not, ask if they know who in the area does.

Reader's Guide to Periodical Literature

The Reader's Guide was the standard index to general periodicals before the new high tech devices were developed. This guide, which is updated six times each year, lists periodicals by subject. It is limited primarily to general interest publications so professional and technical journal articles will not be included. However, most of the articles that are indexed are articles geared to a general audience so they are quite understandable.

Accessing the Reader's Guide to Periodical Literature

This index is available at most general libraries including smaller community libraries.

Index Medicus

This is essentially an index to articles in the field of medicine worldwide. It is a massive several volume guide updated every two months. Articles are indexed by subject, and in a separate volume, by author.

My own feeling is that Index Medicus is decidedly more difficult and time consuming to use than the computerized databases are and that computer databases yield better results. Nevertheless, if you don't have access to the computerized databases in this chapter, or if you are more comfortable doing research the old fashioned way, Index Medicus was the standard before computerized databases were developed.

Accessing Index Medicus

This index is readily available at medical libraries and at some larger general libraries.

Medline

Medline is a computerized database citing about 6.6 million articles from approximately 3,600 biomedical journals published in the United

States and abroad. About 80% of the citations included are to English language items. All citations included in Index Medicus are included here. Medline is updated weekly except during November and December when it is updated monthly. About 30,000 citations are added each month. About 70% of the citations include a good abstract (summary) of the article being cited.

You can search Medline by subject including by up to 4 keywords, by author, title or partial title, and, to some degree, by date.

Medline is an excellent source for the latest information about your illness and treatment options. Recent studies, including results from clinical trials are available here. This is different from PDQ which includes information on clinical trials taking place, but does not normally include results of those trials.

Much of the material found in Medline is very technical and can be overwhelming to the lay person. To fully understand it, you will probably want your physician to help you in interpreting it. Information gleaned from Medline can be very valuable in learning about new treatments and in deciding which treatment is best for you to pursue.

Note that the Cancerlit database discussed below, contains every Medline entry that is cancer related, and some information not found in Medline. Therefore, if you use Cancerlit, there is no need to also use Medline.

Accessing Medline

Medline is only available via computer. Here are a few ways to access it.

Medlars
Medlars (described above) is an excellent vehicle for accessing Medline. Grateful Med or Medlars command language can be used.

CompuServe
You can also access Medline through CompuServe through a reseller called Paperchase. This reseller has put together a reasonably user friendly menu driven access system for searching Medline. To access

Paperchase and through it Medline via CompuServe type "GO PAPERCHASE" at any prompt. It is a CompuServe premium service which means it carries additional charges.

Dialog

Medline is also available through Dialog (file 155 for 1966 to present) and Knowledge Index (file MEDI1). Dialog offers a menu option for searching Medline, or it can be accessed using Dialog command language. Note that Dialog commands differ from Medlars commands.

Medical Libraries

Many medical libraries have access to Medline on-line, on CD-ROM, or both. As with PDQ access, library policies differ as to allowing patron access, but those with CD-ROM are more likely to allow you to search on your own or to help you search for appropriate information.

SDIline

SDIline is a database that contains only the most recent month's updates for Medline. At the end of each month, the entire database is replaced with the references entered into Medline during that month. This service is very useful for anyone with an illness who wants to be current on developments. Of course, it is important to check Medline or Cancerlit at least once before using SDIline or else you will miss everything that came before the most current month. Note that SDIline includes only Medline entries; it does not include entries specific to Cancerlit.

Accessing SDIline

SDIline is available through Medlars. Like Medline, it can be accessed by using either Medlars command language or the Grateful Med software package. You can in fact set up the search criteria and save it so that it can be run every month for each month's updates.

Cancerlit

This Medlars database includes journal articles, government reports, papers, thesis, and other information about virtually every type of cancer. It includes, but is not limited to, all cancer references found in Medline. Therefore, using this database makes using Medline unnecessary for cancer related information gathering.

Some of the items that are not from Medline involve findings from outside the U.S.. However, most of the Cancerlit citations are for English language items. More than 70% of the items derived from Medline include abstracts, as do all the non-Medline items.

This database is updated monthly.

Accessing Cancerlit

Cancerlit is only available via computer.

Medlars
Medlars (described above) is an excellent vehicle for accessing Cancerlit. Either Medlars command language or Grateful Med can be used to access Cancerlit.

Dialog
Cancerlit is also available through Dialog (file 159) and Knowledge Index (file MEDI10). Dialog offers access through a menu option, or through Dialog's command language.

Embase

This medical database (formerly called Excerpta Medica) is owned and operated by Elsevier Science Publishers in Amsterdam, Holland. Although similar to Medline, it has a more complete collection of information about non-U.S. research, especially that involving drugs and drug based therapy.

If you are looking for a foreign clinical trial or information about a drug agent not yet available for use in the U.S., this database is well worth a try.

Embase does have a few problems when used by individuals in search of information on their own illnesses. First, it is very expensive to use. The cost is significantly lower if you access it through Dialog's after hour service, Knowledge Index (see below). Second, to make full use of the database you need to know its command language. While it does offer a menu use option, this mode of use restricts you in what you can do and the limitations you can place on retrieving information. You run the risk of getting more information than you want, and paying more because of it. There simply is no user friendly software of the caliber of Grateful Med (for Medlars) for Embase searching.

If you know the Embase command language or Dialog's command language, you have far more flexibility in using Embase. You can, for example, limit your search to clinical trials only, specific country journals, or specific languages.

Accessing Embase

Embase is only available via computer.

Dialog
Of the services discussed in this section, only Dialog and its evening and night service, Knowledge Index, offers access to Embase. It is less expensive to use through Knowledge Index. Dialog file 72 includes 1985 to present and file 73 includes 1974 to present. On Knowledge Index, file MEDI3 includes 1982 to present. Dialog offers both a menu driven option for Embase and a command language version.

Embase is also available through a few specialized database vendors not discussed here. However, if you have access to BRS, Data-Star, or STN, you will find it there as well.

CD-ROM
Currently, Embase is available on CD-ROM on a limited basis. The company makes several CDs for different areas of medicine, one of which is a cancer CD. It includes references and abstracts from several journals going back to 1982, but it is not as inclusive as the Embase on-line service.

The Embase Cancer CD is new as of this writing, so its availability is limited. Eventually, major medical libraries can be expected to subscribe to Embase on CD-ROM.

National Organization for Rare Disorders (NORD)

NORD is a non-profit organization dedicated to identifying, controlling, and curing rare or orphan diseases. It includes information such as overviews, new treatments, and sources of further information for many rare (and some not-so-rare) cancers. The organization is largely supported by pharmaceutical companies so not surprisingly, most of the treatments are drug based.

NORD is certainly worth checking, especially if your's is a relatively rare illness. The rarer the illness the less likely it is that a physician will be versed in it's current treatment unless that physician specializes in the condition. NORD may be able to point you in the direction of valuable information.

Accessing NORD

CompuServe
NORD's database can be searched on-line through CompuServe (type "GO NORD" from any prompt). It is a relatively easy to use menu driven database that is available without charge beyond CompuServe's basic fees. At this writing, there is no on-line access to the database other than through CompuServe.

By Mail
If your illness is included in NORD's database, you can get a report by mail directly from the association. Currently, the first report is free. Additional reports cost $3.25.

National Organization for Rare Diseases
P.O. Box 8923
New Fairfield, CT 06812
(203) 746-6518

CATline

This Medlars database contains citations for virtually all titles cataloged in the National Library of Medicine Collection. Entries are for meetings, symposiums, articles, and even audiovisual materials. This database is updated weekly. A little more than half the citations refer to non-English language items.

Citations include an NLM reference number. While all referenced items are ultimately available from the NLM, access is another matter. There is a hierarchical system for obtaining documents from the NLM. First, try a local medical library. If they don't have it, they can request it from an NLM regional office and ultimately from the NLM if necessary. However, they will not necessarily do this on behalf of a patient without affiliation to its parent organization (the hospital or medical school that controls the library).

Some documents may be obtained from a Federal Depository Library (see chapter two). Be sure to bring the NLM reference number with you.

There is a Medlars database called DOCUSER that provides information on over 12,000 medical and health libraries worldwide (11,000 of which are in the U.S.) including NLM interlibrary lending policies. Unfortunately, you can't use this database unless you know NLM's command language. However, the librarian at your local medical library may have access, know the language, and be willing to search for you.

Physician's Desk Reference (PDR)

This is the profession's standard directory to drugs, including chemotherapy agents. It is updated and published annually.

PDR lists and cross references available drugs by their manufacturer, product name, and generic and chemical name. It includes a comprehensive description of each drug along with its appropriate use and proper dosage and administration.

It also describes situations where each drug should not be used (where it is contraindicated), various warnings and precautions, and possible adverse reactions and side effects.

Checking out the drug that your physician is proposing in PDR is certainly a judicious and relatively easy precaution.

Accessing Physician's Desk Reference

General Libraries
Physician's Desk Reference is available at larger general libraries. Less current issues may be available at smaller community libraries.

Medical Libraries
Any decent medical library will have a copy of the latest edition of this guide.

Physician's Office
Most physicians keep a current edition of Physician's Desk Reference in the office. However, it is not usually intended for patient use. Few physicians make it available to patients the way they so readily make *Time, Newsweek,* or *People* available.

Chapter Conclusion

Your doctor's treatment proposal may be the best there is for you in your situation. Then again, it may not be. Basic research, such as that outlined in chapter two, and a second opinion from a major research center will cut down the likelihood that you will receive less than the best treatment available. The more extensive kind of research proposed in this chapter will minimize the chance that your treatment will be any less effective and less safe than the best currently available.

The well known cancer surgeon and author Dr. Bernie Siegel categorizes those patient with the best survival skills and survival prospects as exceptional patients. To be an exceptional patient according to Dr. Siegel, you must become an expert in your own illness. If you carry out the kind of research discussed in this chapter you will become that expert. ❖

CHAPTER NINE

❖

Having the Research
Done For You

As this book neared completion, I asked several people to read it and to give me their candid reactions and criticisms. There was one problem that several of my readers mentioned. They complained that for some one without computer experience, using on-line databases can be a real struggle. While all the readers were convinced that on-line databases were essential to getting the latest information, several thought I was underestimating the difficulty involved in learning to use these databases. One doctor who read the manuscript said, "I'm sure to you searching by computer is not all that complicated because you've been using computers for years. I haven't, and I think it would be harder for one of my patients or for myself to learn than you make it out to be." He also pointed out that he doubts many of his patients have open access to computers, modems, and the requisite software.

Other readers had similar comments. While on-line searching is not complicated to people familiar with using computerized databases, I now understand that most people have no such familiarity. I also understand that some one just diagnosed with a life threatening illness has more than enough to worry about without adding the rigors of learning a new computer skill. Further, the people who are interested in taking steps to assure their doctor is not overlooking important new information are, by nature, the same people who do not want to take the chance of omitting an important article because they are not experienced at on-line searching.

Schine On-line Services

In essence, my readers convinced me that patients faced with a serious illness need a service that would do for them, the kind of research I advocate. To that end, I set-up Schine On-line Services.

Through this company, my researchers and I gather information on any and all types of cancer or other serious illness directly for clients. Everyone working as a researcher (including myself) has on-line search experience and training from the National Library of Medicine and from Embase. We can search the databases for you and provide a report of the current findings and clinical trials for your type of illness.

Comprehensive Reports

Our comprehensive reports include:

❖ A lay-person overview of your illness (from PDQ)
❖ A technical overview of your illness (from PDQ physician Section)
❖ A listing of current clinical trials for your illness, including contact names for participating doctors (from PDQ)
❖ Latest findings from Cancerlit
❖ Latest findings from Embase
❖ Latest findings from The National Organization for Rare Disorders (NORD) if available
❖ A list of medical libraries in your state for follow up research

A typical report for cancer is between 90 and 180 pages, and for non-cancer illnesses between 50 and 120 pages. Compiling a report currently costs $179.00.

Monthly Updating Service

If there is one thing I hope this book makes clear, it is that new developments in medicine are taking place all the time. It is not an exaggeration to say that next month or the month after a new development that can save your life may be reported, but by the time your doctor learns of it, it may be too late. For this reason, we also offer a monthly updating service.

At the beginning of each month, we check the latest month's entries to Cancerlit or SDIline, and check clinical trials added to PDQ.

All relevant findings and new clinical trial information is promptly mailed to every client subscribing to the updating service.

Special Research Services

Over the few short months that Schine On-line has been in business we have been asked to do a good deal of specialized research for our clients. Some of the requests included:

❖ I want to know what you can find out about a chemotherapy protocol called CHOP.

❖ Has my doctor even been sued or disciplined by the state medical board?

❖ Has splenectomy been used effectively to combat Non Hodgkins Lymphoma?

❖ What treatments were common for breast cancer before 1990?

❖ How can I get into a certain clinical trial that my doctor doesn't know about?

We try to accommodate all special research requests. Call and ask us about specialized searching.

Doing Your Own Research
Versus Having it Done For You

Previous chapters of this book contain all the information you need to do you own research. If you are versed in using computers and on-line databases, or you want to take the time to learn these skills, there is no reason that you can not retrieve the same information we can. The databases we use are all outlined in the previous chapter.

If you do not have the necessary equipment or the experience in on-line searching, it would be quicker, cheaper, and more efficient to have us do it for you. We know how to get what we are searching for efficiently while minimizing the chances of serious omissions. Our charge for compiling a comprehensive report and for the monthly updating service is fixed so you don't need to worry about running up large on-line bills.

To Reach Us

If you are interested in having us do on-line searching for you or want more information about our search services contact me right away. I will be happy to discuss our services with you. ❖

Schine On-line Services
39 Brenton Avenue
Providence, RI 02906
(800) FIND CURE   (800) 346-3287
(401) 751-3320

CHAPTER TEN

❖

Conclusion

Perhaps there is no more trusted institution in this country than the institution of medicine. It is accepted as fact that health care in this country is first-rate, at least for those with the means to pay the bill. Yet few of us could answer the question, "What are the criteria for the best care?"

So many of us assume that every physician licensed to practice medicine is up to date on the latest developments in his field. That assumption is as naive as it is comfortable. Physicians simply are not required to be up on all the latest developments. While some are current, others adhere loyally to the technology and practices they learned years ago and look skeptically, if at all, upon life saving advances.

Too many cancer (and other) patients get less than the best care available. Yet it is not fair to place the burden of blame for this problem solely with physicians. Most are hard working and highly skilled professionals with busy schedules. Few have the time to do research for patients. Further, physicians hold different opinions and philosophies as to the preferred degree of aggressiveness. Some are quite conservative preferring to stay with the tried and true. Others are willing to be more aggressive; to take calculated risks in the hope of better outcomes.

You as a patient need to educate yourself about your own illnesses so you can become a sophisticated consumer of medicine; so you can participate in saving your own life. First you must learn the basics of your illness and its treatment options. If you don't learn these basics, you can not make decisions based on knowledge; you can not even ask your doctor the right questions. If there are choices to made on the conservative to aggressive spectrum, you should make them based on your own philosophies and needs combined with your new understanding of your illness. If there are new treatments in clinical trial, you must take responsibility for finding out about them and their appropriateness for your situation.

To get the best there is, you have to know what the options are. You need to ask your doctor about those options and demand answers based on science, not based on personal bias or sacred cow beliefs. You need to research your illness through the independent sources that I have described. Finally and above all else, you need to get at least one independent opinion from a physician who is expert in your illness. Finding and seeing that expert is not as daunting a task as it seems if you are prepared to be aggressive and use the procedures outlined in chapter 6.

There was a time in our history when many institutions successfully restricted information and kept decision making out of the hands of its consumers. Schools used to vehemently argue that parents should not have access to their children's records because they would not understand them and such access would create havoc in the system. Today the law guarantees such access to parent. Men in government once argued that women were not capable of understanding the complexities of government and therefore should not have the right to vote. This argument in fact prevailed until 1920. Thanks to the suffragettes, we now understand that this principle was folly.

Today, medicine is one of the few institutions that still tries to keep information and decision making out of the hands of its consumers. Obstacles are erected to keep us from our own records because "we won't understand them" or because "a little knowledge is a dangerous thing." The kind of information gathering that I advocate is frowned upon because "patients won't understand the technical information." Paradoxically, medical information is more readily available than information in most other fields thanks to myriads of publications and electronic databases designed for practitioners but available to anyone. The patients who insist upon using the resources to gather information may well get better medical treatment than the others.

Americans can get the best care in the world but we do not get it automatically. Many will get second best because they do not have the information they need to get any better than that. By becoming a sophisticated consumer and your own expert, you can make sure you know what the best is, and you can make sure that you get it. ❖

❖

Epilogue

It has been just about a year since I started this book. It is my fourth book and my first on this topic (all the others were about small business). This is by far my most important book and the only one for which I wish there was no need.

Since starting the book, I have received enthusiastic encouragement from people with cancer, people who love someone with cancer, and people who have no such tragedy in their life but understand that some day they might.

I continue to do well as a survivor. Now, two and a half years from my diagnosis and nearly two years from treatment, I am cancer free and more than ever expect to remain so. Even though the CAT scans, bone marrow biopsies, and IVs are years behind me, not a day goes by that I don't think about how fearful I was, and how lucky I am to be alive and healthy.

I hope that you too can be as fortunate as I am. I hope that you too can some day look back on your illness as something that was, not something that is. And I hope that the experience helps you to better appreciate life as it certainly did for me. ❖

APPENDIX I
Glossary

These are some of the words used by health professionals in describing cancer, medical conditions and situations relating to cancer, human organs, and cancer treatment. For a more complete list of relevant words and definitions, consult a medical dictionary.

Active immunity: Immunity produced by the body in response to stimulation by a disease-causing organism or a vaccine.

Acute lymphocytic leukemia: A disorder of blood cell production in which abnormal white blood cells accumulate in the blood and bone marrow. (Also called acute lymphatic leukemia and acute lymphoblastic leukemia.)

Adenoids: Masses of lymphatic tissue behind the nose. If enlarged, they may obstruct breathing.

Adjuvant therapy: A treatment method used in addition to the primary therapy. Radiation therapy is often used as an adjuvant to surgery.

Agammaglobulinemia: An almost total lack of immunoglobulins, or antibodies.

Alopecia: The loss of hair from the body and/or the scalp.

Anemia: Low red blood cell count; symptoms include shortness of breath, lack of energy, and fatigue.

Anesthesia: A procedure in which a patient receives medications that block out pain.

Angiogram: An x-ray of the blood vessels.

Anorexia: Absence or loss of appetite for food.

Antibody: A substance, probably made by lymphocytes and certain other specialized cells, which helps defend the body against infections due to viruses, bacteria, and other foreign organisms.

Antibody-dependent-cell-mediated-cytotoxicity (ADCC): An immune response in which antibody, by coating target cells, makes them vulnerable to attack by immune cells.

Antiemetic: A medicine to prevent or relieve nausea and vomiting.

Antigens: Chemical structures in a cell which can be recognized by a patient as foreign and thus stimulate immune reactions.

Antinuclear antibody (ANA): An autoantibody directed against a substance in the cell's nucleus.

Antiserum: Serum that contains antibodies.

Antitoxins: Antibodies that interlock with and inactivate toxins produced by certain bacteria.

Autoantibody: An antibody that reacts against a person's own tissue.

Autoimmune disease: A disease that results when the immune system mistakenly attacks the body's own tissues. Rheumatoid arthritis and systemic lupus erythematosus are autoimmune diseases.

Bacterium: A microscopic organism composed of a single cell. Many but not all bacteria cause disease.

Basophil: A white blood cell that contributes to inflammatory reactions. Along with mast cells, basophils are responsible for the symptoms of allergy

B cells: Small white blood cells crucial to the immune defenses. Also known as B lymphocytes, they are derived from bone marrow and develop into plasma cells that are the source of antibodies.

Benign tumor: A growth that is not cancer and does not spread to other parts of the body.

Biological response modifiers: Substances, either natural or synthesized, that boost, direct, or restore normal immune defenses. BRMs include interferons, interleukins, thymus hormones, and monoclonal antibodies.

Biological therapy: Treatment by stimulation of the body's immune defense system.

Biopsy: The removal of a sample of tissue and examination of it under the microscope to see if cancer cells are present.

Biotechnology: The use of living organisms or their products to make or modify a substance. Biotechnology includes recombinant DNA techniques (genetic engineering) and hybridoma technology

Bladder: The body's reservoir for urine. It is located in front of the rectum.

Blast cells: An immature stage in cellular development before appearance of mature cells.

Blood Count: The number of red blood cells, white cells, and platelets in a given sample of blood.

Bone marrow: The marrow is the spongy material which fills the cavities of the bones and is the substance in which many of the blood elements are produced. In order to determine the condition of the marrow, a doctor may take a small sample from one of the bones in the chest, hip, spine, or leg. The bone marrow is the source of all blood cells.

Brachytherapy *(BRAK-ee-THER-ah-pee):* Treatment with radioactive sources placed into or very near the tumor or affected area; includes surface application, body cavity application (intracavitary), and placement into the tissue (interstitial). Sometimes this term is used interchangeably with "internal radiation therapy."

Cancer: A general term for about 100 diseases characterized by abnormal and uncontrolled growth of cells. The resulting mass, or tumor, can invade and destroy surrounding normal tissues. Cancer cells can spread through the blood or lymph to start new cancers in other parts of the body.

Carcinogen: Any agent that is known to cause cancer.

Catheter: A tube used for injection or withdrawal of fluid.

Cell: The basic structure of living tissues; all plants and animals are made up of one or more cells.

Cellular immunity: Immune protection provided by the direct action of immune cells (as distinct from soluble molecules such as antibodies).

Central nervous system: The brain and spinal cord together form the body's central nervous system. The brain controls body functions by receiving and transmitting messages along a network of nerves that extend throughout the body. The messages reach the brain through the spinal cord.

Cervix: The lower, narrow end of the uterus.

Chemotherapy: Treatment with anticancer drugs.

Chromosomes: Physical structures in the cell's nucleus that house the genes. Each human cell has 23 pairs of chromosomes.

Clinical trial: A study conducted with human patients to determine the effectiveness and safety of a new treatment. Before a treatment is used in clinical trial, it is first tested with animals. When first used with humans, it is administered only to those who would not be helped with standard treatments.

Clone: A group of genetically identical cells or organisms descended from a single common ancestor, or, to reproduce multiple identical copies.

Cobalt 60: A radioactive substance used as a radiation source to treat cancer.

Colon: The lower 5 to 6 feet of the intestine. Also called the large bowel.

Combination chemotherapy: The use of several drugs at the same time or in a particular order to treat cancer.

Complement: A complex series of blood proteins whose action "complements" the work of antibodies. Complement destroys bacteria, produces inflammation, and regulates immune reactions.

Complement cascade: A precise sequence of events, usually triggered by an antigen-antibody complex, in which each component of the complement system is activated in turn.

Constant region: That part of an antibody's structure that is characteristic for each antibody class.

CT scan or **CAT scan:** Computed tomography. An X-ray test that uses a computer to produce a detailed picture of a cross-section of the body.

Cytokines: Powerful chemical substances secreted by cells. Cytokines include lymphokines produced by lymphocytes and monokines produced by monocytes and macrophages.

Cytotoxic T cells: A subset of T lymphocytes that can kill body cells infected by viruses or transformed by cancer.

Dietitian: A specialist in nutrition and diet counseling.

Dosimetrist *(do-SIM-uh-trist):* A person who plans and calculates the proper radiation dose for treatment.

Endometrium: The lining of the uterus

Eosinophil: A white blood cell that contains granules filled with chemicals damaging to parasites, and enzymes that damp down inflammatory reactions.

Epitope: A unique shape or marker carried on an antigen's surface, which triggers a corresponding antibody response.

Erythrocytes: Red blood cells. They use hemoglobin, to carry oxygen as it is breathed in through the lungs to all parts of the body.

External radiation therapy: A type of cancer treatment that uses a machine to focus high-energy rays on the cancer site.

Gamma rays: Same as x-rays but from a different radioactive source.

Gastrointestinal (GI): Having to do with the digestive tract, which includes the stomach and the intestines.

Gene: A unit of genetic material (DNA) that carries the directions a cell uses to perform a specific function, such as making a given protein.

Graft-Versus-Host Disease (GVHD): A life-threatening reaction in which transplanted immunocompetent cells attack the tissues of the recipient. GVHD is a potential danger in bone marrow transplants.

Granulocytes: White blood cells filled with granules containing potent chemicals that allow the cells to digest microorganisms, or to produce inflammatory reactions. Neutrophils, eosinophils, and basophils are examples of granulocytes.

Granulocytopenia: A term indicating a deficiency of granulocytes in the blood.

Gray: A measurement of absorbed radiation dose; I gray = 100 rads.

HL-A: Human histocompatibility antigens. These antigens appear on white blood cells as well as cells of almost all other tissues and are analogous to red blood cell antigens (A, B, etc.). By typing for HL-A antigens, donors and recipients of white blood cells, platelets, and organs can be "matched" to insure good performance and survival of transfused and transplanted cells.

Hemorrhage: A general term for loss of blood brought about by injury to the blood vessels or by a deficiency of certain necessary blood elements such as platelets.

Helper T cells: A subset of T cells that typically carry the T4 marker and are essential for turning on antibody production, activating cytotoxic T cells, and initiating many other immune responses.

Histocompatibility testing: A method of matching the self antigens (HLA) on the tissues of a transplant donor with those of the recipient. The closer the match, the better the chance that the transplant will take.

Hormone therapy: Treatment of cancer by removing or adding hormones.

Human leukocyte antigens (HLA): Protein in markers of self used in histocompatibility testing. Some HLA types also correlate with certain autoimmune diseases.

Humoral immunity: Immune protection provided by soluble factors such as antibodies, which circulate in the body's fluids or "humors," primarily serum and lymph.

Hybridoma: A hybrid cell created by fusing a B lymphocyte with a long-lived neoplastic plasma cell, or a T lymphocyte with a lymphoma cell. A B-cell hybridoma secretes a single specific antibody.

Hyperfractionated radiation: Division of the total dose of radiation into smaller doses that are given more than once a day.

Hypogammaglobulinemia: Abnormally low levels of immunoglobulins.

Immune complex: A cluster of interlocking antigens and antibodies.

Immune system: The complex group of cells and organs that defend the body from foreign substances that might cause infection or disease.

Immune response: The reactions of the immune system to foreign substances.

Immunoassay: A test using antibodies to identify and quantify substances. Often the antibody is linked to a marker such as a fluorescent molecule, a radioactive molecule, or an enzyme.

Immunocompetent: Capable of developing an immune response.

Immunoglobulins: A family of large protein molecules, also known as antibodies.

Immunosuppression: Reduction of the immune responses, for instance by giving drugs to prevent transplant rejection.

Immunotherapy: See biological therapy

Immunotoxin: A monoclonal antibody linked to a natural toxin, a toxic drug, or a radioactive substance.

Infusion: The process of putting fluids into the vein by letting them drip slowly through a tube.

Injection: The use of a syringe to "push" fluids into the body; often called a "shot."

Interleukins: A major group of lymphokines and monokines.

Internal radiation: A type of therapy in which a radioactive substance is implanted into or close to the area needing treatment. (See also *interstitial implant and intracavitary implant.*)

Interstitial implant: A radioactive source placed directly into the tissue (not in a body cavity).

Intracavitary implant: A radioactive source placed in a body cavity such as the chest cavity or the vagina.

Intramuscular (IM): Into a muscle: some anticancer drugs are given by IM injection.

Intraoperative radiation: A type of external radiation used to deliver a large dose of radiation therapy to the tumor bed and surrounding tissue at the time of surgery

Intravenous (IV): Into a vein; anticancer drugs are often given by IV injection or infusion.

LAK cells: Lymphocytes transformed in the laboratory into lymphokine-activated killer cells, which attack tumor cells.

Langerhans cells: Dendritic cells in the skin that pick up antigen and transport it to lymph nodes.

Larynx: The upper part of the windpipe. The larynx produces the voice and is also called the voice box.

Leukemia: A cancer of the blood forming organs (bone marrow, spleen).

Leukocytes: All white blood cells.

Linear accelerator: A machine that creates and uses high-energy x-rays to treat cancers.

Liver: An organ in the body which performs many complex functions necessary for life. These include processes related to digestion, production of certain blood proteins, and elimination of many of the body's waste products.

Local treatment: Treatment that affects cells in the tumor and the area close to it.

Lymph: A transparent, slightly yellow fluid that carries lymphocytes, bathes the body tissues, and drains into the lymphatic vessels.

Lymph nodes: Small, bean-shaped organs that filter harmful materials such as bacteria; located throughout the body in places such as the neck, underarm, and groin.

Lymphatic system: A chain of organs, including lymph nodes, that carries lymph fluids throughout the body; makes and stores cells that fight infection.

Lymphatic vessels: A bodywide network of channels, similar to the blood vessels, which transport lymph to the immune organs and into the bloodstream.

Lymphocytes: Small white blood cells produced in the lymphoid organs and paramount in the immune defenses.

Lymphoid organs: The organs of the immune system, where lymphocytes develop and congregate. They include the bone marrow, thymus, lymph nodes, spleen, and various other clusters of lymphoid tissue. The blood vessels and lymphatic vessels can also be considered lymphoid organs.

Lymphokines: Powerful chemical substances secreted by lymphocytes. These soluble molecules help direct and regulate the immune responses.

Macrophage: A large and versatile immune cell that acts as a microbe-devouring phagocyte, an antigen-presenting cell, and an important source of immune secretions.

Major histocompatibility complex (MHC): A group of genes that controls several aspects of the immune response. MHC genes code for self markers on all body cells.

Malignant: Cancerous. Used to describe a tumor made up of cancerous cells.

Mammogram: An x-ray of the breast.

Mast cell: A granule-containing cell found in tissue. The contents of mast cells, along with those of basophils, are responsible for the symptoms of allergy

Melanoma: A rare type of cancer of the cells that produce melanin (pigment in the skin). Melanoma usually begins in the skin, often as a mole that is dark in color. Unlike the common skin cancers, melanoma tends to spread to internal organs.

Menopause: The time in a woman's life when regular menstruation permanently stops, usually between the ages of 45 and 55; also called "change of life."

Metastasis: The spread of cancer from the original tumor to another part of the body. Cells in the metastatic tumor (secondary tumor) are the same as those in the original cancer.

Microbes: Minute living organisms, including bacteria, viruses, fungi, and protozoa.

Microorganisms: Microscopic plants or animals.

Monoclonal antibodies: Antibodies produced by a single cell or its identical progeny, specific for a given antigen. As a tool for binding to specific protein molecules, monoclonal antibodies are invaluable in research, medicine, and industry.

Monocyte: A large phagocytic white blood cell which, when it enters tissue, develops into a macrophage.

Monokines: Powerful chemical substances secreted by monocytes and macrophages. These soluble molecules help direct and regulate the immune responses.

Natural killer (NK) cells: Large granule-filled lymphocytes that take on tumor cells and infected body cells. They are known as " natural" killers because they attack without first having to recognize specific antigens.

Neoplasm: Abnormal cell growth of tissue. See cancer.

Neutrophils: A type of white blood cell that plays a major role in the body's defense against bacteria, viruses, and fungi.

OKT3: A monoclonal antibody that targets mature T cells.

Oncologist: A physician who is a specialist in the treatment of cancer.

Opportunistic infection: An infection in an immunosuppressed person caused by an organism that does not usually trouble people with healthy immune systems.

Ovary: The female reproductive organ in which eggs are formed. The female hormone estrogen also comes from this organ.

Palliative therapy: A treatment that may relieve symptoms without curing the disease.

Pancreas: An organ of the digestive system located behind the stomach. The pancreas secretes chemicals that help digest food. It also secretes insulin, which changes blood sugar into sources of quick energy.

Passive immunity: Immunity resulting from the transfer of antibodies or antiserum produced by another individual.

Pathologist: A doctor who studies cells and tissues to determine if a disease is present.

Pelvis: The lower part of the abdomen located between the hip bones.

Phagocytes: Large white blood cells that contribute to the immune defenses by ingesting microbes or other cells and reign particles.

Pharynx: The throat; specifically, the upper part of the throat just behind the mouth.

Plasma cells: Large antibody-producing cells that develop from B cells.

Platelet: One of the main components of the blood. Forms clots that seal up injured areas and prevent hemorrhage.

Platelet-pheresis: A process in which platelets are removed from normal whole blood by centrifugation.

Polymorph: Short for polymorphonuclear leukocyte or granulocyte.

Polyp: A growth of mucous membrane that bulges into a cavity of the body, such as the colon or nose.

Precancerous: A term used to describe a condition that may or is likely to become cancer.

Prostrate: A gland of the male reproductive system that lies just below the bladder and surrounds part of the canal that empties the bladder.

Prosthesis: An artificial replacement for a missing body part such as an artificial limb or breast form.

Rad: Short form for "radiation absorbed dose;" a measurement of the amount of radiation absorbed by tissues (100 rad = 1 gray).

Radiation: Energy carried by waves or a stream of particles.

Radiation implant: A small container of radioactive material that is placed in or near a cancer.

Radioactive isotopes: Substances that give off radiation. Used in small amounts to diagnose cancer.

Radiation oncologist: A doctor who specializes in using radiation to treat cancer.

Radiation therapist: A person with special training who runs the equipment that delivers the radiation. Sometimes called a "radiation technologist."

Radiation therapy: Treatment using high-energy radiation from X-ray machines, radium, cobalt, or other sources.

Radiologist: A physician with special training in reading diagnostic x-rays and performing specialized x-ray procedures.

Radiotherapy: See radiation therapy.

Recurrence: Reappearance of cancer at the same site (local), near the initial site (regional), or in other areas of the body (metastatic).

Red blood cells: Cells that carry oxygen to all the various organs and tissues of the body.

Remission: The decrease or disappearance of a cancer and its symptoms. Also the period during which this occurs.

Scavenger cells: Any of a diverse group of cells that have the capacity to engulf and destroy foreign material, dead tissues, or other cells.

Screening: Using tests to find disease when there are no symptoms.

Scrotum: The pouch that contains the testicles.

Serum: The clear liquid that separates from the blood when it is allowed to clot. This fluid retains any antibodies that were present in the whole blood.

Side effects: Problems caused when cancer treatment affects healthy cells in the body. Common side effects are fatigue, nausea, vomiting, decreased blood cell counts, and mouth sores.

Sigmoidoscope: A tubelike instrument used to examine part of the colon.

Simulation: A process involving special x-ray pictures that are used to plan radiation treatment so that the area to be treated is precisely located and marked for treatment.

Spleen: Abdominal organ which performs a function similar to that of lymph nodes in that it acts as a filter. It frequently becomes enlarged in leukemia.

Stage: The extent of disease; how doctors classify whether cancer has spread from its original site to another part of the body.

Stem cells: Cells from which all blood cells derive. The bone marrow is rich in stem cells.

Stomatitis: Sores on the inside lining of the mouth.

Stool: The matter discharged in a bowel movement.

Subunit vaccine: A vaccine that uses merely one component of an infectious agent, rather than the whole, to stimulate an immune response.

Superantigens: A class of antigens, including certain bacterial toxins, that unleash a massive and damaging immune response.

Suppressor T Cells: A subset of T cells that turn off antibody production and other immune responses.

Surgery: An operation.

Systemic treatment: Treatment that reaches and affects cells everywhere in the body (such as chemotherapy, hormone therapy, and biological therapy).

T Cells: Small white blood cells that orchestrate and/or directly participate in the immune defenses. Also known as T lymphocytes, they are processed in the thymus and secrete lymphokines.

Teletherapy: Treatment in which the radiation source is at a distance from the body. Linear accelerators and cobalt machines are used in teletherapy.

Testicles: The two eggshaped glands that are located in the scrotum. Also called the testes, these glands are part of the male reproductive system and secrete male hormones.

Thymus: A primary lymphoid organ, high in the chest, where T lymphocytes proliferate and mature.

Thyroid gland: A gland that produces hormones responsible for growth and metabolism. It is located near the upper part of the trachea (windpipe).

TIL (Tumor infiltrating lymphocytes): These immune cells are extracted from the tumor tissue, treated in the laboratory, and reinjected into the cancer patient.

Tissue typing: See histocompatibility testing.

Toxins: Agents produced by plants and bacteria, normally very damaging to mammalian cells, that can be delivered directly to target cells by linking them to monoclonal antibodies or lymphokines.

Treatment port: The place on the body at which the radiation beam is aimed.

Tumor: An abnormal mass of tissue that results from excessive cell division. Tumors perform no useful body function. They may be either benign (not cancer) or malignant (cancer).

Ultrasound: A method to diagnose disease that bounces high-frequency sound waves off tissue and changes the echoes into pictures.

Uterus: The hollow organ in which the unborn child develops until birth; also called the womb.

Vaccine: A substance that contains antigenic components from an infectious organism. By stimulating an immune response (but not disease), it protects against subsequent infection by that organism.

Variable Region: That part of an antibody's structure that differs from one antibody to another.

Vagina: The muscular canal that leads from the uterus to the outside of the body; also called the birth canal.

White blood cells: The blood cells responsible for fighting infection. The two types of white blood cells are called granulocytes and lymphocytes.

X-Rays: High-energy radiation used in high doses to treat cancer or in low doses to diagnose the disease.

APPENDIX II
NCI Designated Cancer Centers

National Cancer Institute
Comprehensive and Clinical Cancer Centers

A single asterisk (*) indicates a comprehensive cancer center and a double asterisk (**) indicates a clinical cancer center. See chapter six for an explanation of NCI designated comprehensive and clinical care centers.

Information about referral procedures, treatment costs, and services available to patients can be obtained from the individual cancer centers listed below.

ALABAMA
University of Alabama at Birmingham
Comprehensive Cancer Center*
Basic Health Sciences Building, Room 108
1918 University Boulevard
Birmingham, AL 35294
Telephone (205) 934-6612

ARIZONA
University of Arizona Cancer Center*
1501 North Campbell Avenue
Tucson, AZ 85724
Telephone (602) 626-6372

CALIFORNIA
The Kenneth T. Norris Jr.
Comprehensive Cancer Center*
University of Southern California
1441 Eastlake Avenue

Los Angeles, CA 90033-0804
Telephone (213) 226-2370

Jonsson Comprehensive Cancer Center*
University of California at Los Angeles
200 Medical Plaza
Los Angeles, CA 90027
Telephone (310) 206-0278

City of Hope National Medical Center**
Beckman Research Institute
1500 East Duarte Road
Duarte, CA 91010
Telephone (818) 359-8111, ext. 2292

University of California at San Diego Cancer Center**
225 Dickinson Street
San Diego, CA 92103
Telephone (619) 543-6178

COLORADO
University of Colorado Cancer Center**
4200 East 9th Avenue, Box B190
Denver, CO 80262
Telephone (303) 270-7235

CONNECTICUT
Yale University Comprehensive Cancer Center*
333 Cedar Street
New Haven, CT 06510
Telephone (203) 785-6338

DISTRICT OF COLUMBIA
Lombardi Cancer Research Center*
Georgetown University Medical Center
3800 Reservoir Road, N.W.
Washington, DC 20007
Telephone (202) 687-2192

FLORIDA
Sylvester Comprehensive Cancer Center*
University of Miami Medical School
1475 Northwest 12th Avenue
Miami, FL 33136
Telephone (305) 548-4800

ILLINOIS
University of Chicago Cancer Research Center**
5841 South Maryland Avenue
Chicago, IL 60637
Telephone (312) 702-9200

MARYLAND
The Johns Hopkins Oncology Center*
600 North Wolfe Street
Baltimore, MD 21205
Telephone (410) 955-8638

MASSACHUSETTS
Dana-Farber Cancer Institute*
44 Binney Street
Boston, MA 02115
Telephone (617) 732-3214

MICHIGAN
**Meyer L. Prentis Comprehensive Cancer Center of
Metropolitan Detroit***
I10 East Warren Avenue
Detroit, MI 48201
Telephone (313)745-4329

University of Michigan Cancer Center*
101 Simpson Drive
Ann Arbor, MI 48109-0752
Telephone (313) 936-9583

MINNESOTA
Mayo Comprehensive Cancer Center*
200 First Street Southwest
Rochester, MN 55905
Telephone (507) 284-3413

NEW HAMPSHIRE
Norris Cotton Cancer Center*
Dartmouth-Hitchcock Medical Center
2 Maynard Street
Hanover, NH 03756
Telephone (603) 646-5505

NEW YORK
Memorial Sloan-Kettering Cancer Center*
1275 York Avenue
New York, NY 10021
Telephone 1-800-525-2225

Columbia University Comprehensive Cancer Center*
College of Physicians and Surgeons
630 West 168th Street
New York, NY 10032
Telephone (212) 305-6905

Roswell Park Cancer Institute*
Elm and Carlton Streets
Buffalo, NY 14263
Telephone (716) 845-4400

Albert Einstein College of Medicine**
Cancer Research Center
Chanin Building
1300 Morris Park Avenue
Bronx, NY 10461
Telephone (212) 920-4826

Kaplan Cancer Center*
New York University Medical Center
462 First Avenue
New York, NY 10016-9103
Telephone (212) 263-6485

University of Rochester Cancer Center**
601 Elmwood Avenue, Box 704
Rochester, NY 14642
Telephone (716) 275-4911

NORTH CAROLINA
Duke Comprehensive Cancer Center*
P.O. Box 3814
Durham, NC 27710
Telephone (919) 286-5515

UNC Lineberger Comprehensive Cancer Center*
University of North Carolina School of Medicine
Chapel Hill, NC 27599
Telephone (919) 966-4431

**Cancer Center of Wake Forest University at the
Bowman Gray School of Medicine***
300 South Hawthorne Road
Winston-Salem, NC 27103
Telephone (919) 748-4354

OHIO

Ohio State University Comprehensive Cancer Center*
410 West 10th Avenue
Columbus, OH 43210
Telephone (614) 293-8619

Ireland Cancer Center
Case Western Reserve University**
University Hospitals of Cleveland
2074 Abington Road
Cleveland, OH 44106
Telephone (216) 844-5432

PENNSYLVANIA

Fox Chase Cancer Center*
7701 Burholme Avenue'
Philadelphia, PA 19111
Telephone (215) 728-2570

University of Pennsylvania Cancer Center*
3400 Spruce Street
Philadelphia, PA 19104
Telephone (215) 662-6364

Pittsburgh Cancer Institute*
200 Meyran Avenue
Pittsburgh, PA 15213-2592
Telephone 1-800-537-4063

RHODE ISLAND

Roger Williams Cancer Center**
825 Chalkstone Avenue
Providence, RI 02908
Telephone (401) 456-2071

TENNESSEE
St. Jude Children's Research Hospital**
332 North Lauderdale Street
Memphis, TN 38101-0318
Telephone (901) 522-0306

TEXAS
Institute for Cancer Research and Care**
4450 Medical Drive
San Antonio, TX 78229
Telephone (512) 616-5580

**The University of Texas M.D. Anderson Cancer.
Center***
1515 Holcombe Boulevard
Houston, TX 77030
Telephone (713) 792-3245

UTAH
Utah Regional Cancer Center**
University of Utah Health Sciences Center
50 North Medical Drive, Room 2C10
Salt Lake City, UT 84132
Telephone (801) 581-5052

VERMONT
Vermont Cancer Center*
University of Vermont
1 South Prospect Street
Burlington, VT 05401
Telephone (802) 656-4580

VIRGINIA
Massey Cancer Center**
Medical College of Virginia
Virginia Commonwealth University
1200 East Broad Street
Richmond, VA 23298
Telephone (804) 786-9641

WASHINGTON
Fred Hutchinson Cancer Research Center*
1124 Columbia Street
Seattle WA 98104
Telephone (206) 667-4675

WISCONSIN
Wisconsin Clinical Cancer Center*
University of Wisconsin
600 Highland Avenue
Madison, WI 53792
Telephone (608) 263-8090

APPENDIX III

National Cancer Institute Free Publications

The following booklets and related materials are available without charge from the National Cancer Institute. They can be ordered by calling the NCI Cancer Information Service at 1-800-4-CANCER.

GENERAL MATERIALS

Cancer Information Service Leaflet (1-800-4-CANCER). This leaflet explains the toll-free information system, sponsored by the National Cancer Institute and regional cancer centers, to help the public obtain answers to their questions about cancer.

Lo Que Usted Debe Saber Sobre El Cancer (What You Should Know About Cancer) (83-1828). This bilingual booklet, directed toward people of Hispanic origin, answers questions on cancer causes, prevention, and treatment. Includes glossary. 33 pages.

RESEARCH REPORTS (Series). In-depth reports covering current knowledge of the causes and prevention, symptoms, detection and diagnosis, and treatment of various types of cancer.

Adult Kidney Cancer and Wilms' Tumor (90-2342). (Revised April 1989) 25 pages.
Bone Cancers (91-721). (Revised June 1990) 14 pages.
Bone Marrow Transplantation (92-1178). (Revised April 1991). 29 pages.
Cancer of the Bladder (90-722). (Revised October 1989) 22 pages.
Cancer of the Colon and Rectum (92-95). (Revised October 1991).
Cancer of the Lung (90-526). (Revised July 1989) 23 pages.
Cancer of the Ovary (89-3014). 18 pages.
Cancer of the Pancreas (88-2941). 12 pages.
Cancer of the Prostate (91-528). (Revised September 1990) 21 pages.
Cancer of the Stomach (88-2978). 18 pages.

Cancer of the Uterus: Endometrial Cancer (91-171). (Revised June 1990) 15 pages.

Leukemia (88-329). (Revised November 1987) 20 pages.

Melanoma (89-3020). 22 pages.

Oral Cancers (92-2876). (Revised November 1991).

Skin Cancers: Basal Cell and Squamous Cell Carcinomas (91-2977). (Revised September 1990) 17 pages.

Understanding The Immune System. (92-529). (Revised October 1991) This pamphlet describes the complex network of specialized cells and organs that make up the human immune system. It explains how the system works to fight off disease caused by invading agents such as bacteria and viruses, and how it sometimes malfunctions, resulting in a variety of diseases from allergies, to arthritis, to cancer. It was developed by the National Institute of Allergy and Infectious Diseases and printed by the National Cancer Institute. 40 pages.

WHAT YOU NEED TO KNOW ABOUT CANCER. This series of pamphlets discusses symptoms, diagnosis, treatment, emotional issues, and questions to ask the doctor. Includes glossary of terms and other resources.

Cancer (90-1566) (Revised August 1988)
Bladder (91-1559)(Revised June 1989)
Bone (90-1571)(Revised April 1990)
Brain & Spinal Cord (90-1558)
Breast (91-1556)(Revised May 1989)
Cervix (90-2047)(Revised April 1990)
Colon and Rectum (90-1552)(Revised December 1987)
Dysplastic Nevi (91-3133)
Esophagus (91-1557)
Hodgkin's Disease (90-1555)(Revised August 1988)
Kidney (91-1569)
Larynx (90-1568)
Adult Leukemia (88-1572)
Childhood Leukemia (91-1573)
Lung (91-1553)(Revised August 1987)
Melanoma (90-1563)(Revised September 1988)
Multiple Myeloma (90-1575)

Non-Hodgkin's Lymphoma (90-1567) (Revised November 1988)
Oral Cancers (91-1574) (Revised June 1989)
Ovary (91-1561) (Revised May 1990)
Pancreas (90-1560) (Revised October 1989)
Prostate (90-1576) (Revised April 1990)
Skin (90-1564) (Revised August 1988)
Stomach (90-1554)
Testis (88-1565) (Revised June 1988)
Uterus (91-1562) (Revised August 1988)

Facts On Cancer Sites (Revised May 1987). Spanish versions of some of the *What You Need To Know About Cancer* pamphlets.
Cervix
Colon and Rectum
Lung
Mouth
Prostate
Stomach
Uterus

PATIENT MATERIALS

ANTICANCER DRUG INFORMATION SHEETS IN SPANISH/ENGLISH. These sheets on 30 of the most common anticancer drugs have been developed for Spanish-speaking cancer patients. Each sheet provides information about side effects, proper usage, and precautions. These sheets, a useful accompaniment to "Tratamiento de Quimoterapia Para El Cancer," were prepared by the United States Pharmacopeial Convention, Inc., for distribution by NCI.

Asparginasa/Asparaginase
Bleomicina/Bleomycin
Busulfano/Busulfan
Carmustina/Carmustine
Ciclofosfamida/
Cyclophosphamide
Cisplatin/Cisplatin
Citarabina/Cytarabine

Clorambucilo/Chlorambucil
Dacarbazino/Dacarbazine
Dactinomicina/Dactinomycin
Daunorrubicina/Daunorubicin
Doxorrubicina/Doxorubicin
Estreptozocina/Streptozocin
Estramustina/Estramustine
Floxiridina/Floxuridine

Hidroxiurea/Hydroxyurea	Plicamicina/Plicamycin
LomustinaLomustine	Prednisona/Prednisone
Mecloretamina/Mechlorethamine	Procarbazina/Procarbazine
Melfalano/Melphalan	Tamoxifeno/Tamoxifen
Mercaptopurina/Mercaptopurine	Vinblastina/Vinblastine
Metotrexato/Methotrexate	Fluorouracilo/Fluorouracil
Mitomicina/Mitomycin	Vincristina/Vincristine
Mitotano/Mitotane	

Advanced Cancer: Living Each Day (87-856). This booklet addresses living with a terminal illness, how to cope, and practical considerations for the patient, the family, and friends. 30 pages.

BREAST CANCER PATIENT EDUCATION SERIES

BREAST BIOPSY: WHAT YOU SHOULD KNOW (90-657). (Revised December 1989) This booklet discusses biopsy procedures, what to expect in the hospital, awaiting the diagnosis, and coping with the possibility of breast cancer. 16 pages.

Breast Cancer: Understanding Treatment Options (91-2675). (Revised June 1990) This booklet summarizes the biopsy procedure, types of breast surgery (giving advantages and disadvantages for each), radiation therapy as primary treatment, adjuvant therapy and making treatment decisions. 19 pages.

Mastectomy: A Treatment For Breast Cancer (91-658). (Revised June 1990) This booklet presents information about the different types of breast surgery, what to expect in the hospital and during the recovery period, and coping with having breast surgery. Breast self-examination for mastectomy patients is also described. 25 pages.

Radiation Therapy: A Treatment For Early Stage Breast Cancer (91-659). this booklet discusses the treatment steps (surgery and radiation therapy), possible side effects, precautions to take after treatment, and emotional adjustment to having breast cancer. 20 pages.

After Breast Cancer: A Guide To Followup Care (90-2400). This booklet is for the woman who has completed treatment. It explains the importance of continuing breast self examination, regular physical exams, possible signs of recurrence, and managing the physical and emotional side effects of having had breast cancer. 15 pages.

Breast Reconstruction: A Matter Of Choice (91-2151). (Revised June 1990) This booklet discusses the techniques used in reconstructive breast surgery, possible complications, answers to common questions, criteria for choosing a plastic surgeon, and issues of emotional adjustment. 21 pages.

Cancer Treatments: Consider The Possibilities (89-3060). This easy to read brochure is designed to make patients aware of clinical trials as a treatment option.

Datos Sobre El Tratamiento De Quimioterapia Contra El Cancer (91-3232S). This flyer in Spanish, provides a brief introduction to cancer chemotherapy.

Chemotherapy And You: A Guide To Self-Help During Treatment (91-1136). (Revised June 1990) This booklet, in question-and answer format, addresses problems and concerns of patients receiving chemotherapy. Emphasis is on explanation and self-help. Includes glossary of terms and an entire section dealing with anticancer drugs and drug combinations. 64 pages.

Eating Hints: Tips And Recipes For Better Nutrition During Cancer Treatment (91-2079). (Revised April 1990) This cookbook-style booklet includes recipes and suggestions for maintaining optimum, yet realistic, good nutrition during treatment. All recipes have been tested. Originally produced by the Yale-New Haven Medical Center and reprinted by the NCI. 96 pages.

Facing Forward: A Guide For Cancer Survivors (90-2424). This booklet presents a concise overview of important survivor issues, including ongoing health needs, psychosocial concerns, insurance, and employment. Easy-to-use format includes real-life survivor experiences, practical tips, record keeping forms, and resources. Recommended for cancer survivors, their family, and friends. 43 pages.

Help Yourself: Tips For Teenagers With Cancer (91-2211). (Revised November 1990) This magazine-style booklet is designed to provide information and support to adolescents with cancer. Issues addressed include reactions to diagnosis, relationships with family and friends, school attendance, and body image. May be used in conjunction with audiotape. Produced in cooperation with Adria Laboratories, Incorporated. 37 pages.

Hospital Days, Treatment Ways (91-2085). (Revised March 1988) This hematology-oncology coloring book helps orient the child with cancer to hospital and treatment procedures. Originally produced by the Ohio State University Comprehensive Cancer Center and Children's Hospital, Columbus, Ohio. 26 pages.

Managing Interleukin-2 Therapy (89-3071). This booklet explains what patients can expect during treatment, possible side effects and management of these symptoms. Questions are included for patients to ask their health care providers while undergoing interleukin-2 treatments. 14 pages.

Managing Your Child's Eating Problems During Cancer Treatment (92-2038). This booklet contains information about the importance of nutrition, side effects of cancer and cancer treatment, ways to encourage your child to eat, and special diets. 32 pages.

Patient To Patient: Cancer Clinical Trials And You. This 15-minute videocassette provides simple information for patients and families about the clinical trials process (produced in collaboration with the American College of Surgeons Commission on Cancer).

Radiation Therapy And You: A Guide To Self-Help During Treatment (91-2227). (Revised October 1990) This booklet addresses concerns of patients receiving external and internal forms of radiation therapy. Emphasis is on explanation and self-help. 52 pages.

El Tratamiento De Radioterapia (92-3239S). This flyer in Spanish, provides a brief introduction to radiation therapy for cancer.

Taking Time: Support For People With Cancer And The People Who Care About Them (91-2059). (Revised June 1990) This sensitively written booklet for persons with cancer and their families addresses the feelings and concerns of others in similar situations and how they have coped. 72 pages.

Talking With Your Child About Cancer (91-2761). (Revised June 1990) This booklet is designed for the parent whose child has been recently diagnosed with cancer. It addresses the health-related concerns of young people of different ages and suggests ways to discuss disease-related issues. 16 pages.

What Are Clinical Trials All About? (90-2706). This booklet is designed for patients who are considering taking part in research for cancer treatment. It explains clinical trials to patients in easy-to-understand terms and gives them information that will help them decide about participating. Includes a glossary. 24 pages.

When Cancer Recurs: Meeting The Challenge Again (90-2709). This booklet details the different types of recurrence, types of treatment, and coping with cancer's return. 28 pages.

When Someone In Your Family Has Cancer (90-2685). (Revised May 1990) This booklet is written for young people whose parent or sibling has cancer. It includes sections on the disease, its treatment, and emotional concerns. Includes a glossary. 28 pages.

Young People With Cancer: A Handbook For Parents (92-2378). (Revised March 1988) This booklet discusses the most common types of childhood cancer, treatments and side effects, and issues that may arise when a child is diagnosed with cancer. Offers medical information and practical tips gathered from the experience of others. A glossary, bibliography, list of reading materials, and fold-out drug chart are included. Developed in cooperation with the Candlelighters Childhood Cancer Foundation. 85 pages.

APPENDIX IV
Associations for Cancer Patients and Survivors

The associations listed in this appendix are involved in cancer research, education, or support for those whose lives are affected by cancer. Most of the information included here was reported directly by each association and was not verified or edited by the author or publisher.

American Association for Cancer Education
401 Community Health Services Building
Birmingham, AL 35294

The American Association for Cancer Education (AACE), founded in 1966, is a professional organization of people from many disciplines who are working to improve the quality of education in the field of neoplastic diseases. It provides a forum for those concerned with the education of health professionals working to advance the prevention of cancer, expedite early cancer detection, promote individualized therapy, and develop rehabilitation programs for cancer patients. The AACE's efforts include the faculties of schools of medicine, dentistry, osteopathy, education, pharmacy, nursing, public health, and social work. The association encourages projects for the training of para-medical personnel and educational programs for the general public, populations at risk, and patients with cancer. Annual meetings of the AACE present innovations in the field and review techniques employed in cancer education from the prevention of cancer to oncology education.

American Cancer Society
1599 Clifton Road, N.E.
Atlanta, GA 30329
TEL (800) ACS-2345

The American Cancer Society (ACS) was originally established as the American society for the control of cancer in 1913, and became the ACS in1945. ACS is the voluntary organization dedicated to eliminating cancer as a major health problem. It conducts and supports programs of research, education, and service to the cancer patient. The society's immediate goal of saving more lives is served through educating the public about prevention and early detection of cancer, the importance of prompt treatment, and the possibilities of cure, through educating the medical profession to the latest advances in diagnosis and treatment of cancer, and through direct service to the cancer patient and the patient's family. Public education activities include publication of a variety of pamphlets, educational programs conducted in schools and communities, and presentation of materials in the mass media. The society has a comprehensive professional education program designed to motivate physicians, dentists, and nurses to use the best cancer management techniques. The society conducts service and rehabilitation programs for cancer patients and their families. ACS supports cancer research through several types of research grants and disseminates the research results. ACS has 57 divisions as well as over 3000 local units.

American Institute for Cancer Research
1759 R Street, NW
Washington, DC 20009
TEL (202) 328-7744; (800)-843-8114

The American Institute for Cancer Research (AICR), a non-profit organization, is dedicated to informing the public on how to reduce the risk of cancer and how to detect the early signs. AICR concentrates on diet and nutrition as methods of cancer control. AICR also supports cancer research grants and sponsors conferences on the role of diet and nutrition in the development and treatment of cancer.

Association for Research of Childhood Cancer
P.O. Box 251
Buffalo, NY 14225-0251
TEL (716) 681-4433

The Association for Research of Childhood Cancer (AROCC) is a nonprofit organization, staffed by volunteers, formed in 1971 by parents who had lost children to pediatric cancer. The seven charter members determinedto raise funds by various projects in order to provide "seed money" to various pediatric research centers in order to find a cure and, ultimately, prevent the types of cancer that attack children. Funds are also obtained from community activities; memorial contributions; and donations from businesses, private foundations, and concerned individuals. As a parent support group AROCC aids parents of young cancer victims by distributing information on treatment, emotional aspects, and patient services via their publications.

Australian Cancer Society, Inc. (ACS)
GPO Box 4708
Sydney, NSW, 2001
Australia
TEL (02) 267-1944
TEL FAX (02) 261-4123

The Australian Cancer Society, Inc. (ACS), is a federation of the independent and autonomous state cancer organizations created to foster national and international cooperation and development of all activities in relation to cancer. The ACS provides national research grants, vacation scholarships, public and professional education programs, submissions at federal level on patient welfare and benefits. The ACS is concerned with all aspects of cancer research, education, and patient welfare services.

Canadian Cancer Society
Societe' Canadienne du Cancer
77 Bloor Street, West
Suite 1702
Toronto, Ontario
Canada, M5S 3A1
TEL (416) 961-7223
TEL FAX (416) 961-4189

The Canadian Cancer Society is a national, community based organization of volunteers, whose mission is the eradication of cancer and the enhancement of the quality of life of people living with cancer. The Canadian Cancer Society achieves its mission through programs of research, education, patient services, fund-raising and influences on public policy. The society consists of a large volunteer membership and small supporting staff which appropriates $25 million toward cancer research and carries out programs of public education. The society offers emotional support programs and services including transportation, drugs, and medical services supplementing those that are provided by the government.

Cancer Federation, Inc.
11671 Sterling, rm. J
Riverside, CA 92503
TEL (714) 359-3794

Cancer Federation promotes research and education in the field of cancer immunology. It encourages development of appropriate cancer therapies using natural biological modifiers. It publishes *Challenge of the Cancer Federation*, a quarterly newsletter on cancer and treatment.

Cancer Care
National Cancer Foundation
1180 Avenue of the Americas
New York, NY 10036
TEL (212) 302-2400

Cancer Care, Inc. is a non-profit social service agency founded in 1944 to help cancer patients and their families and friends cope with the impact of cancer. Cancer Care treats people at all stages of illness and provides help to both patients and families. There are no fees. Cancer Care provides information and referral to homemaking services, hospices, child care services, hospitals, and other community resources; guidance to develop a plan for care for the patient at home; professional counseling for cancer patients and their families, on both an individual basis and in groups; bereavement counseling to help surviving family members cope with the loss of a loved one; supplementary financial assistance to help families meet certain home care costs such as homemakers, home health aides, housekeepers, and for transportation for treatment; a volunteer visitor program for frail or homebound cancer patients; worksite counseling and consultation services to help employers and employees respond to their concerns about cancer; and education and training regarding the psychosocial aspects of cancer for health professionals and allied health care providers.

Cancer Guidance Institute
1323 Forbes Avenue
Suite 200
Pittsburgh, PA 15219
TEL (412) 261-2211

The Cancer Guidance Institute (formerly the Lifeline Institute) is a nonprofit agency specializing in assisting people whose lives have been affected by cancer. The Institute strives to help by offering emotional support and guidance through the course of the illness, by providing information on obtaining a second opinion, by directing local callers to useful community services, and by helping the patient learn positive ways of coping. The organization also offers a 24-hour hotline for the Pittsburgh area, a speaker service, workshops and conferences, as well as several publications on living with cancer. The Institute is funded from corporate and private foundations, memberships, memorials, and individual gifts.

Cancer Hopefuls United for Mutual Support
c/o Dr. Howard Mase
27 Paerdegat Seventh Street
Brooklyn, NY 11236
TEL (718) 251-8456

Cancer Hopefuls United for Mutual Support (CHUMS) was started in 1981 as a national self-help organization emphasizing the quality of life for all who have a history of cancer. Its purpose is to help cancer survivors and their families better understand the disease and cope with the resulting problems. CHUMS offers self-help sessions, crisis intervention services, Phone-a-Patient and Visit-a-Patient programs, sponsorship of research, and house-hotel facilities to ease the financial burdens of patients undergoing treatment. CHUMS is funded by contributions and membership fees.

Cancer Research Center
3501 Berrywood Dr.,
Columbia, MO 65201
Ben W. Papermaster, Ph.D., Director
TEL (314) 875-2255
TEL (314) 875-2256-57 (Women's Cancer Control Program)

The Cancer Research Center is a nonprofit organization. Interests: research in the field of cancer immunotherapy, specifically with the use of lymphokines; research in the area of detection of early cancers, especially breast, colorectal, uterine-cervix, and lung; education of the general public and the health professional about cancer; studies of infectious organisms in the cancer patient. holdings: collection of materials in the above areas. Publications: *Mirror* (quarterly); brochures (numerous titles) on most aspects of cancer patient care, treatment, and rehabilitation, most of which are intended to help patients cope with their diseases and treatments; technical reports, journal articles, state-of-the-art reviews, critical reviews, abstracts, reprints. Information services: answers inquiries; provides educational materials about cancer; conducts seminars; lends materials; makes referrals to other sources of information; permits onsite use of collection. Services are free and available to anyone.

Cancer Research Institute
133 East 58th Street
New York, NY 10022
TEL (800) 223-7874

CRI was founded in 1953 to foster the field of cancer immunology. The organization encourages (sometimes financially through research grants) the exploration of the ability of the body's own immune system to be stimulated to fight cancer. It champions the development of immunotherapies as alternatives and adjuncts to traditional treatments. It publishes a booklet, *Cancer and the Immune System— The Vital Connection*, available for free from the organization.

Cancervive
6500 Wilshire Boulevard.Suite 500
Los Angeles, CA 90048
TEL (213) 203-9232

Cancervive was founded to serve the needs of cancer survivors. Through several local organizations, it sponsors support groups for survivors and generally helps survivors deal with social, employment and work, health insurance, and other problems faced by those with cancer in their past or present.

Candlelighters Childhood Cancer Foundation
1312 18th Street, NW, Suite 200
Washington, DC 20036
TEL (202) 659-5136; (800) 366-CCCF

The Candlelighters Childhood Cancer Foundation, an international organization formed in 1970 as the Candlelighters, consists of 400 local groups of parents whose children have or have had cancer. The Foundation acts as a national coordinator, providing the communications link among the groups through a newsletter and parent correspondence programs. Candlelighters identifies the needs of childhood and adolescent cancer patients and their families, provides guidance in coping with cancer's effects, serves as an emotional support system, and seeks cancer research funding. The organization is also concerned with the quality and availability of information and education materials for parents of children with cancer and for long term survivors.

Children's Cancer Research Institute
2351 Clay Street, Suite 512
San Francisco, CA 94115
TEL (415) 923-3540

The Children's Cancer Research Institute (CCRI) is a non-profit, family-oriented organization devoted to developing improvements in anti-cancer therapy and better supportive care for patients with cancer and their families. CCRI has been directly involved with well over 1,000 infants, children and young adults with cancer and has brought improvements in care to thousands more throughout the world in the past 15 years. To supplement the traditional medical cancer treatments (surgery, chemotherapy and radiation), other programs are offered. These include: direct assistance with transportation and lodging costs and other necessities for needy families, a chaplain, art therapist, summer camp, recreation activities, a family newsletter, and support groups.

Corporate Angel Network
Building One
Westchester County Airport
White Plains, NY 10604
Tel (914) 328-1313

Corporate Angel Network is made up of U.S. corporations that own their own aircraft. Empty seats are offered free to cancer patients (and one attendant) needing transportation to or from treatment facilities. Patient must be able to board plane unassisted, and not need special equipment or services en route.

Dana-Farber Cancer Institute
44 Binney St.
Boston, MA 02115
TEL (617) 732-3487

Introduction: a nonprofit organization partially sponsored by the National Cancer Institute, the institute conducts clinical cancer research and administers cancer control and community outreach projects. Interests: cancer research; interdisciplinary patient care; clinical investigation, including chemotherapy and immunotherapy; supportive patient care, including platelet and granulocyte transfusions; clinical microbiology; drug development and pharmacology; tumor immunology; tumor virology; molecular genetics; cytogenetics; cytokinetics; biostatistics; epidemiology; all growth and regulation; molecular biology; molecular carcinogenesis; pediatric and medical oncology. Holdings: computerized data base with some important information regarding institute patients and the latest ICDA classifications. Publications: journal articles. Information services: answers inquiries; provides advisory services; conducts seminars and workshops; makes referrals to other sources of information. Services are free and available to anyone. Patient information is restricted to nonconfidential data for statistical use only.

Georgetown University
Lombardi Cancer Research Center
3800 Reservoir Rd. NW., Washington, DC 20007
TEL (202) 687-2192

This Comprehensive Cancer Center, part of the National Cancer Institute's national network, is involved in multidisciplinary basic and clinical research. It serves as a resource for cancer diagnosis, treatment, and control, and participates in a national program of cancer data acquisition and analysis. Interests: cancer research, diagnosis, treatment, medical education. Publications: *Lombardi Cancer Center* (newsletter); directories; patient education literature. Information Services: Cancer Information Service (CIS), a center program, answers inquiries, provides advisory services and information on research in progress, evaluates data, distributes publications, and makes referrals to other sources of information. These services are free and available to anyone. The center also conducts free seminars that are restricted to health professionals and provides a free consultation service that is available to medical professionals and patients in the area as well as the greater region.

Independent Citizens Research Foundation for the Study of Degenerative Diseases
P.O. Box 97
Ardsley, NY 10502
TEL (914) 478-1862

The Independent Citizens Research Foundation for the Study of Degenerative Diseases (ICRF) was established to disseminate information on the causes and prevention of chronic illnesses and to underwrite research projects offering an early and practical applicability of the findings to the problems of those afflicted with such illnesses. The foundation reports pertinent research findings with respect to causes, early detection procedures, and possible approaches to therapy and prevention of degenerative diseases. Research projects which could result in findings immediately applicable to the prevention of suffering are supported by the foundation.

International Agency for Research on Cancer (IARC)Library
International Agency for Research on Cancer
150 Cours Albert Thomas
69372 Lyon CEDEX 2, FRANCE
TEL 875.81.81

Agency holdings include over 286 periodicals; about 8,200 books; 8,500 bound volumes of journals; WHO publications; reports; access to the computerized data bases which contain cancer-related data. Publications: IARC issues scientific publications, monographs, and annual reports. A publications list is available. Information services: Answers inquiries; provides advisory, reference, literature-searching, and reproduction services; makes interlibrary loans; permits onsite use of collection. Services are free and available to anyone.

International Association of Cancer Victors and Friends
7740 West Manchester Avenue, Suite 110
Playa del Rey, CA 90293
TEL (213) 822-5032

The International Association of Cancer Victors and Friends (IACVF), formerly known as The International Association of Cancer Victims and Friends, founded in 1963, is an advocacy agency which disseminates educational materials concerning the prevention and control of cancer through the use of nontoxic therapies. Major IACVF concerns are the restoration of the cancer victim's and his family's right to free choice of treatment for cancer and the physician's right to use nontoxic, beneficial therapies for all cancer victims. The Association publishes information relating to cancer-causing factors in the environment, food, and drink; cancer prevention; cancer detection; and nontoxic cancer treatments.

International School for Cancer Care
The Royal Marsden Hospital, Fulham Rd.
London SW3 6JJ, England
Mrs. Gillian V.J. Hunter, Director
TEL (44) 01-376 3623

Introduction: Funded by charitable donations, the International School for Cancer Care is the successor of the World Federation for Cancer Care, now defunct. The International School for Cancer Care facilitates the training of health care workers in the supportive care of all cancer patients, in cancer rehabilitation, extended palliative care and in terminal care. It also promotes the supportive care of the family/ key persons during the patient's illness and in bereavement. Interests:

Palliative cancer care; education of health care workers globally in palliative cancer care. Holdings: Information and materials on cancer patient care; world data base on cancer patient care. Publications: *Newsletter 1988.* Information services: Sponsors health care workers at international meetings and for work experience; conducts seminars and workshops; facilitates hospice projects, especially in developing countries.

International Union of Immunological Societies
c/o Dr. Henry Metzger, Secretary-General
9650 Rockville Pike
Bethesda, MD 20814
TEL (301) 530-7178

Immunology; immunochemistry; cellular immunology; allergy; microbial immunology; organ transplants; cancer immunology; standardization of immunodiagnostic reagents, nomenclature, and educational activities. Publications: Booklet describing the Union's activities. Information services: Answers inquiries; provides advisory services; makes referrals to other sources of information. Services are free and available to anyone.

Leukemia Society of America
Communications Department
733 Third Avenue
New York, NY 10017
TEL (212) 573-8484

The Leukemia Society of America, founded in 1949 as the deVilliers Foundation, funds individual researchers seeking cures for leukemia and other diseases of the blood-forming tissues, provides financial aid to leukemia patients, and conducts educational programs aimed at the public and health care professionals. Public education is conducted through seminars, media presentations, and publications. Professional education efforts include seminars, symposia, and publications covering developments in treatment. Patients may apply to local chapters for financial aid. The society has 57 chapters, which serve as local support groups.

Linus Pauling Institute of Science and Medicine (LPI)
440 Page Mill Rd.
Palo Alto, CA 94306
TEL (415) 327-4064

The institute is partially sponsored by the federal government and private foundations. Interests: Research in 3 interrelated fields of cancer, aging, and nutrition. In regard to cancer, most studies bear on nutritional prevention and control of cancer and on molecular and viral mechanisms of carcinogenesis. In many of the studies, including those on aging, quantitative protein profiling by 2-dimensional gel electrophoresis is one of the technologies that has been widely applied and developed. Holdings: Small research library of about 800 volumes (books and journals); access to the Dialog computerized data bases. Publications: *Cancer and Vitamin C* (book, 1979); journal articles, bibliographies, data compilations, reprints. A publications list is available. Information services: Answers inquiries and distributes publications. Services are free and available to anyone within limits of time and staff.

M.D. Anderson Cancer Center
Research Medical Library
Box 99
1515 Holcombe
Houston, TX 77030
TEL (713) 792-2282

Interests: Oncology; cancer chemotherapy; radiobiology; pathology; biochemistry; pharmacology; toxicology; anesthesiology; surgery; gynecology; anatomy; histology; cytology; chemistry; electron microscopy; biology; physics; nursing. Holdings: 43,000 volumes; 1,200 current journal subscriptions. Also, *The History of Cancer* collection contains approximately 600 items related to cancer medicine and quackery. An attempt has been made to purchase exhaustively in cancer medicine from the 16th to the 20th Century. The Library has access to multiple data bases, including a locally mounted five-year Medline file. Information services: Answers inquiries; provides reference and duplication services; makes interlibrary loans; permits onsite reference by university faculty and students, Texas residents, and visiting scholars.

Make Today Count
101 1/2 South Union Street
Alexandria, VA 22314
TEL (703) 548-9674

Make Today Count (MTC), founded in 1974, provides self-help support groups in nearly 200 communities throughout the U.S. for patients with cancer and other life-threatening illness, their families, and the professionals who work with them. MTC is a nonprofit organization supported by individual contributions, newsletter subscriptions and gifts. Monthly meetings are provided by each chapter, where members are encouraged to share their experiences in living with life-threatening illness.

McGill University
Faculty of Medicine
McGill Cancer Centre
Faculty of Medicine, McGill University
McIntyre Medical Sciences Bldg.,
Montreal, Quebec, CANADA H3G 1Y6
3655 Drummond St.
TEL (514) 398-3535

Introduction: An integral facility of the Faculty of Medicine, the centre is funded primarily by the National Cancer Institute of Canada and the Medical Research Council of Canada. Interests: Molecular biology of DNA replication and gene amplification in animal cells; molecular genetics of tumor specific cell surface antigens in human cancer; cancer cell surface glycoproteins; cell biology of human tumors; control of differentiation of leukemic and normal hemotopoietic cells. Publications: Books, journal articles, state-of-the-art reviews, critical reviews, abstracts, indexes, reprints. Information services: Provides directions and information for cancer patients; provides advisory services; answers inquiries; conducts seminars and workshops; analyzes data; distributes publications. Services are free and available to anyone.

Memorial Cancer Research Foundation of Southern California, Inc.
1125 South Beverly Dr., Suite 610
Los Angeles, CA 90035
TEL (213) 277-4634

Partially funded by federal money through the National Surgical
Adjuvant Breast Project, Pittsburgh, Pa., and private donations, the
foundation is involved in investigational protocol studies in the
treatment of cancer. Interests: Cancer research; investigational
protocols; breast examination training; investigational treatment
multimodality resources, including surgery, radiation therapy,
chemotherapy, immunotherapy, and hormonal therapy. Holdings:
The foundation is responsible for tumor registry duties at local
hospitals. Collected data is reported to the Cancer Surveillance
Network, headquartered at the University of Southern California.
Information services: Answers inquiries free.

Michigan Cancer Foundation
Leonard N. Simons Research Library
110 East Warren
Detroit, MI 48201
TEL (313) 833-0710

All fields of cancer-related research and associated methods and
techniques; all aspects of cancer diagnosis and therapy; patient and
family counseling; public education. Holdings: 3,000 books; 110
periodical titles; online access to the Dialog, Medline, Cancerline,
Toxline, and protein identification Resource (PIR) computerized data
bases. Publications: Staff research is reported in various scientific
journals. Information services: Answers inquiries; provides reference
services; makes referrals to other sources of information; makes
interlibrary loans. Extensive services are provided only to staff
members.

National Alliance of Breast Cancer Organizations
1180 Avenue of the Americas, 2nd floor
New York, NY 10036
TEL (212) 719-0154

NABCO is made up of several hospitals, research facilities, and other organizations concerned with detection and treatment of breast cancer. It serves as a resource for organizations needing information about breast cancer programs and medical advances. It also disseminates information on health insurance reimbursement, educational materials, and breast cancer support groups. It publishes *NABCO News*, a quarterly newsletter that monitors developments in breast cancer prevention and treatment.

National Coalition for Cancer Survivorship
1010 Wayne Avenue, 5th floor
Silver Spring, MD 20910
TEL -(301) 650-8868

NCCS helps cancer survivors (defined as anyone with a history of cancer) to lead productive and fulfilling lives. It encourages peer support, communications and discussion of issues related to survivorship. It also disseminates information designed to help and support survivors. Finally, NCCS acts as a coordinator for a network of groups, services, and events for cancer survivorship.

National Foundation for Cancer Research, Inc. (NFCR)
7315 Wisconsin Ave. NW.
Suite 332W
Bethesda, MD 20814
TEL (301) 654-1250
Introduction: A nonprofit organization, NFCR conducts basic science cancer research at some 40 laboratories in many nations. Multinational and multidisciplinary, it supports innovative and cutting edge basic science cancer research projects. Interests: All areas of basic science cancer research to include: chemistry; biochemistry; biophysics; physiology; quantum biology; molecular and cellular biology; genetics. Publications: Annual report. Information services: Conducts seminars, workshops, and conferences; evaluates scientific data; provides information on NFCR research in progress; distributes publications; makes referrals to other sources of information. Services are free and available to anyone.

National Leukemia Association, Inc.
Patient Aid Services Director
585 Stewart Avenue, Suite 536
Garden City, NY 11530
TEL (516) 222-1944

The association raises funds on the national level to provide financial
aid for the medical expenses of leukemia patients and funds research
to help find the causes of and cures for leukemia. Patient financial aid
is available for drugs, lab fees, blood, X-ray therapy, and other
expenses not covered by insurance. Service limitations: Patients
applying for aid must submit applications and letters of diagnosis
from their doctors.

Northwestern University
Cancer Center
Communications Program
303 East Chicago Ave.
McGaw Pavilion,
Chicago, IL 60611
TEL (312) 908-5260

Partially sponsored by the National Cancer Institute, the program
integrates and coordinates cancer and cancer-related research and
activities of Northwestern University and affiliated hospitals of the
McGaw Medical Center. It seeks to increase the amount of information and effectively disseminate it to designated target audiences by
developing and formalizing appropriate vehicles of communication.
Interests: Cancer and cancer-related research; oncology; neoplastic
disease. Holdings: Small collection of reprints of publications by
Cancer Center members; collection of current oncological and medical
journals and texts. Publications: *Cancer Focus* (semiannual); biennial
report, research summaries, data compilations, reprints. Information
services: Answers inquiries; provides advisory, consulting, and
reference services; conducts seminars and workshops; provides
information on research in progress; distributes publications; makes
referrals to other sources of information; permits onsite use of collections. Services are free and available to anyone.

Ohio State University
Cancer Center
410 West 12th Ave., Suite 302
Columbus, OH 43210
TEL (614) 422-1382

Sponsored in part by the National Cancer Institute, the Center seeks to translate its own and other laboratories' observations into applicable clinical usage and to communicate existing and newly-developed therapies, diagnostic procedures, and prevention methods throughout the Ohio Valley Lake Erie Region. Interests: Clinical and scientific research into cancer prevention, diagnosis, treatment, knowledge, and care; cancer rehabilitation; cancer etiology; broad-based fundamental laboratory research in these areas. Holdings: Library of pamphlets concerning various aspects of cancer diagnosis, prevention, cure, and rehabilitation; statistical data; small cancer-related library. Publications: Books, journal articles, reprints, physicians' newsletter, professional education pamphlets. Information services: Answers inquiries via Cancer Information Service toll-free telephone number; conducts community outreach to hospitals and physicians regarding cancer treatment, care, and diagnosis; evaluates data; distributes publications and datacompilations; makes referrals to other sources of information. The above services are available to anyone and are free, except for publications, mailing costs, and extensive services requiring labor, supplies, or computer time. Access is available to the following computerized data bases via the Health Sciences Library for a small charge: Medline, AVline, Cancerline, Cancer Proj, Chemline, Serline, and Toxline.

R.A Bloch Cancer Foundation
Cancer Hot Line
R. A. Bloch Cancer Support Center
Cancer Connection
4410 Main St.
Kansas City, MO 64111
TEL (816) 932-8453

Cancer Hot Line is a volunteer organization organized to help cancer patients make necessary decisions in order to have the best chance of beating cancer as easily as possible. Cancer Connection is sponsored by the H&R Bloch Foundation. Interests: Cancer; cancer education; cancer patients; support groups; medical second opinion Publications: *Cancer... There's Hope* and *Fighting Cancer* (both books by Richard and Annette Bloch). Information services: Answers inquiries; makes referrals to other competent sources. Services are free and available to anyone.

Reach to Recovery
(American Cancer Society)
1599 Clifton Rd., N.E.
Atlanta, GA 30329
TEL (404) 320-3333

Reach to Recovery is a short term peer-visitor program sponsored by ACS for women who have or had breast cancer. Volunteers visit at the request of patients' physicians, to help with emotional, physical, and cosmetic needs.

Resource Information Network for Cancer (RINC)
c/o American Cancer Society
2975 Wilshire Blvd., Suite 200
Los Angeles, CA 90010
TEL (213) 386-7660

RINC is a cooperative program of the American Cancer Society, Jonsson Comprehensive Cancer Center, Harbor-UCLA Medical Libraries, and the Los Angeles County Public Library System. Its goal is to establish a library-based network as a means of providing the public in the Los Angeles area with centralized access to current information, materials, and educational programs relevant to cancer control. Interests: Cancer materials and resources. Holdings: Special cancer collections maintained in selected libraries in the Los Angeles County Public Library System. Information services: Answers inquiries; provides advisory and reference services; makes referrals to other sources of information. Services are free and available to anyone within limits of staff time.

St. Jude Children's Hospital
P.O. Box 318
Memphis, TN 38101
TEL (901) 522-0300

The Hospital is partially sponsored by the American Lebanese Syrian Associated Charities. Interests: Basic and clinical research on catastrophic diseases of children with special emphasis on cancer; cancer treatment and rehabilitation; cancer control. Holdings: 2,000 books; 285 journal subscriptions; 9,000 bound volumes; access to NLM Medlars and Dialog. Publications: Annual report, journal articles, reprints. Information services: Answers inquiries; conducts seminars and workshops; makes interlibrary loans; distributes publications. Patients are accepted only by referral from a physician. Consultations are provided only to physicians. All medical services and consultations, including hospitalization, are provided without charge to the patient and, except for consultations, are available to pediatric patients with a catastrophic disease under active study, primarily cancer in its many forms.

Skin Cancer Foundation
245 Fifth Avenue, Suite 2402
New York, NY 10016
TEL (212) 725-5176

SCF provides grants to researchers and offers public education programs. Most programs deal with prevention of skin cancer. It publishes *Melanoma Letter*, a quarterly newsletter on advances in prevention and treatment of skin cancer.

Spirit and Breath Association
8210 Elmwood Avenue, Suite 209
Skokie, IL 60077
TEL (312) 673-1384

Spirit and Breath offers moral and physical support to people with lung cancer and their families, in order to help patients lead normal and productive lives. It serves as a forum for exchanging information among individuals who are (and were) undergoing treatment for lung cancer. It publishes *Spirit and Breath Association Bulletin* a monthly newsletter for lung cancer patients.

Susan G. Komen Foundation
6820 LBJ Fwy. Suite 130
Dallas, TX 75240
TEL (214) 980-8841

This foundation is dedicated to increasing the recovery and survival rates of breast cancer patients. It sponsors research and conducts educational programs.

People's Medical Society
462 Walnut Street
Allentown, PA 18102
TEL (800) 624-8773, (215) 770-1670

People's Medical Society works for and advocates for consumer medical rights. It publishes numerous books, booklets, and newsletters designed to explain consumer rights and to help consumers get the best care possible. Some of its publications deal with cancer treatment, access to medical records, choosing a doctor, and more. Membership is open to anyone.

United Cancer Council, Inc. (UCC)
650 East Carmel Dr., Suite 340
Carmel, IN 46030
TEL (317) 844-6627

Cancer, including service to cancer patients and their families, public and professional education regarding cancer, and applied cancer research. Holdings: An audiovisual library is maintained for member agencies. Publications: *Coordinator* (quarterly); pamphlets. Information services: answers inquiries; provides advisory and other information services to member agencies; distributes educational pamphlets.

University of Hawaii
Cancer Research Center of Hawaii
1236 Lauhala St.
Honolulu, HI 96813
TEL (808) 548-8415

The center is one of the Specialized Cancer Centers in the United States named under the Cancer Act of 1971. A research institute of the University of Hawaii, it conducts a comprehensive program of research in epidemiology, basic science, clinical science, and cancer prevention and control. Interests: Nutritional factors in cancer epidemiology, molecular and cell biology of carcinogenesis, clinical trials and provision of technical support of clinical trials in the community, and cancer prevention and control research. Holdings: computerized tumor registry with statewide data from 1960 and a dedicated computing facility with a computerized population database from 1942, including the capability of constructing family profiles over two to three generations. Publications: Technical reports, journal articles, data compilations. A publications list is available. Information services: Answers questions from the public about the center's activities; conducts seminars for health professionals through the University of Hawaii; operates a cancer communications network and cancer information line; distributes data computations to professionals concerned with cancer. Services are generally provided free.

University of New Mexico
Cancer Center
New Mexico Tumor Registry (NMTR)
900 Camino de Salud NE.
Albuquerque, NM 87131
TEL (505) 277-5541

Located at the UNM Medical Center, the NMTR is supported by grants from the National Cancer Institute and State of New Mexico. Interests: Population-based cancer data for the state of New Mexico and the American Indian populations in Arizona. Holdings: Computerized data base on cancer incidence and mortality within the NMTR area of coverage from 1969 to the present. Publications: *New Mexico Tumor Registry Newsletter*; reports, journal articles, bibliographies, data compilations. Information services: Answers inquiries; conducts seminars; evaluates data; lends materials; distributes publications; permits onsite use of data. Services are free, except for computer time, and available within restrictions imposed by need for confidentiality of certain data.

University of North Carolina at Chapel Hill
School of Medicine
Lineberger Cancer Research Center
School of Medicine - CB 7295
University of North Carolina
Chapel Hill, NC 27599-7295
TEL (919) 966-3036

Sponsored by the National Cancer Institute and the State of North Carolina, the Center seeks an interdisciplinary approach to cancer research by drawing on the resources of the Schools of Medicine, Public Health, Dentistry, Pharmacy, and Nursing, as well as the Departments of Biology and Chemistry. Its goals are to provide research of an outstanding nature; to extend research methods to the benefit of patients; and to implement curriculum programs through various academic departments. Interests: Cancer research; viral oncology; cancer cell biology; immunology; carcinogenesis; drug pharmacology; cancer epidemiology; clinical cancer research; cancer prevention and control; cancer data base; biotechnology. Publications: *Cancer Research Center News*; directories. Information services: Answers inquiries; provides advisory and reference services; provides information on research in progress; evaluates data; conducts seminars and symposia; distributes publications; makes referrals to other sources of information. Services are free, except for laboratory work, and available to anyone.

University of Wisconsin-Madison
Wisconsin Clinical Cancer Center
Department of Human Oncology
Division of Prevention and Quantitative Oncology
Wisconsin/Iowa Cancer Information Service
c/o Wisconsin Clinical Cancer Center
1300 University Ave., 7C
Madison, WI 53706
TEL (608) 262-0046
TEL (800) 422-6237 (in Wisconsin and Iowa)

The Service is funded by the National Cancer Institute. Interests: Any cancer-related topic. Holdings: Materials on cancer; automated Physicians' Data Query (PDQ) database. Publications: *Current Practice Letter.* Information services: Provides answers to questions about cancer and cancer-related services in Wisconsin to the public and health professionals in Wisconsin and Iowa via toll-free phone.

We Can Do!
1800 Augusta, Suite 150
Houston, TX 77057
TEL (713) 780-1057

We Can Do! is made up of a support system of cancer patients and professional psychologists. Its primary purpose is to address the psychological needs of patients and to encourage survivors to provide moral support to cancer patients. It does not answer medical questions but does encourage patients to become involved in their own treatment. It sponsors weekly educational sessions and encourages relaxation, laughter, and positive attitude as adjunct therapy. It offers pamphlets and audio tapes.

Whedon Cancer Foundation
P.O. Box 683
Sheridan, WY 82801
TEL(307) 672-2941
TEL (FAX) (307) 672-7273

Early cancer detection (serological, epidemiological). Holdings: Cancer patient education file of pamphlets for distribution; , ICRDB Cancergram; access to Medline And Docline. Publications: journal articles, activity reports. Information services: answers inquiries; provides advisory and consulting services; conducts research; makes referrals to other sources of information. Cancer searches are available to health care professionals only. Its laboratory facilities are available to patients by physician referral only. Other services are free and available to anyone.

Y-Me National Organization for Breast Cancer Information and Support
18220 Harwood Avenue
Homewood, IL 60430
TEL (708) 799-8338

Y-Me provides peer support and information to women who have breast cancer, as well as presurgical counseling and referral services. It publishes *Breast Cancer Bibliography* (annual) and *Guidelines for Breast Cancer Support Groups.*

APPENDIX V
Selected References

The following publications, mentioned in this book, might be useful to understanding your condition and treatment possibilities. Also, see appendix III for an extensive listing of publications available for free from the National Cancer Institute.

DeVita, Vincent T. Jr., Hellman, Samuel, and Rosenberg, Steven A. *Principles and Practice of Oncology.* J.B. Lippincott Company. Philadelphia Pennsylvania, 1988.

Directory of Medical Specialties. Marquis Who's Who- MacMillan Directory Division. Wilmette, Illinois, updated every two years.

Note: Oncologists are listed under *internal medicine* category.

Encyclopedia of Associations. Gale Research, Detroit, Michigan. (published annually)

Index Medicus. National Institute of Health. Bethesda, Maryland, updated monthly (subject index and author index)

Moossa, A.R., et al. editors, *Comprehensive Textbook of Oncology,* second edition, Williams and Wilkins. Baltimore, Maryland, 1991.

Pinkney, Cathey and Pinckney, Edward R. *The Patient's Guide to Medical Tests.* Facts on File Publications. New York, 1982

Physician's Desk Reference. Medical Economics Company. Oradell, New Jersey, updated annually.

Questionable Doctors. Public Citizen Health Research Group. Washington, D.C. 1991 (updated annually).

Note: The full book currently costs $50.00 for consumers. However, you can buy it on a state by state basis. Current pricing for

the first state section purchased is $12.00 and each additional state section is $5.00. To order:
Public Citizen Health Research Group
2000 P. Street NW
Washington D.C. 20036
202-833-3000

Schlesser, Jerry L. *Drugs Available Abroad- A Guide to Therapeutic Drugs Available and Approved Outside the United States*. Darwent Publications Ltd. and Gale Research. Detroit Michigan, 1990.

Note: According to the publisher, a new edition is scheduled for publications in 1993, and annually thereafter. The 1990 edition is indexed only by name of drug. I suggested, as apparently have several others, that the next edition be indexed by illness. I hope the suggestion is heeded because it would make the publication much more usable.

Wittes, Robert E. MD, *Manual of Oncologic Therapeutics*. J.B. Lippincott Company. Philadelphia Pennsylvania, 1992.

MAGAZINE

Coping Magazine. Michael D. Holt. 2019 North Carothers, Franklin, Tennessee 37064. This is a quarterly magazine designed for people living with cancer.

MEDICAL DICTIONARIES

Medicine has an extensive technical vocabulary. To decipher technical reports and your own records, a good medical dictionary will be extremely useful. Note also that appendix I contains a limited glossary of medical terms primarily related to cancer.

Anderson, Kenneth, N., Anderson, Lois, E., *Mossby's Pocket Dictionary of Medicine, Nursing, and Allied Health*. The C.V. Mossby Company, Saint Louis, Missouri, 1990.

Note: Mossby's Pocket Dictionary is highly recommended. It is understandable to the lay person without being overly simplistic.

Darland's Pocket Medical Dictionary, 24th edition, W.B. Saunders Company- Harcourt, Brace, and Javonich. Philadelphia, Pennsylvania, 1989.

Stedman's Pocket Medical Dictionary, Williams and Wilkins. Baltimore, Maryland, 1987.

Index

L

laetrile 44
Leukemia Society of America 12, 131
libraries
  and access to Medline 77
  Federal Depository 11
  for medical consumer 56
  general 55
  hospital 55
  medical 55
  medical school 56
  National Cancer Institute
    Cancer Information Service 56
  state departments of health 56
Linus Pauling Institute of Science and Medicine (LPI) 132
Lombardi Cancer Research Center 129

M

M.D. Anderson Cancer Center 132
Make Today Count 133
malpractice 22
Manual of Oncologic Therapeutics 13
markers 17
McGill University 133
medical records 24-30
  access to 26
  and monitoring your condition 25
  and the American Medical Association 26
  and the law pertaining to 26, 27
  and tracking your progress 25
  how to obtain yours 27-29
  interpreting 30
  where they are 25
  why you need yours 24
medical textbooks 13
Medlars, see National Library of Medicine
Medline 70, 75
  access 76
    Knowledge Index 77
Memorial Cancer Research Foundation of Southern California Inc. 134
Michigan Cancer Foundation 134